SHORT CASES IN PAEDIATRICS

This book is dedicated to

Maggie and Nilar for their support and encouragement.
A special thanks is due to Gemma Cade for her artwork which has been used on the back cover.

SHORT CASES IN PAEDIATRICS

Authors

ALAN CADE MB ChB DCH MRCP MRCPCH

Lecturer in Paediatrics
University of Leeds
Department of Paediatrics
and Child Health
Leeds, UK

DONALD HODGE BSc(Hons) MBChB MRCP MRCPCH

Lecturer in Paediatrics
University of Leeds
Department of Paediatrics
and Child Health
Leeds, UK

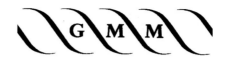

© 2000
Greenwich Medical Media Limited
137 Euston Road
London
NW1 2AA

ISBN 1 84110 009 9

First published 2000

Visit our website at:
www.greenwich-medical.co.uk

Typeset by Phoenix Photosetting Ltd, Chatham, Kent
Printed in China

CONTENTS

Section 1   Examination techniques

Section 2   Short cases

Preface

You are possibly about to take the last professional examination you will take in your life! Getting through the paediatric MRCPCH short case section of the 'part 2 membership' means that unless you perform badly in the rest of the exam you will almost certainly succeed. This last hurdle will make or break you as a person and as a paediatrician. This is the section you are mostly likely to fail in. There is over £400 riding on this 30 minutes of sheer purgatory. This is the opportunity to escape from the drudgery of baby checks, phlebotomy and coffee-making duties to the dizzy heights of 'SpR-ship' and a better life!!

With such huge self-imposed pressure placed upon your weary shoulders, is it small wonder that so many people come unstuck? However, it need not be like that. For those who are well prepared and well versed in the exam and the foibles of the examiners, the short cases can be an almighty anti-climax. At the end of it all a common feeling expressed is 'what on earth was all the fuss about . . . I really found it quite enjoyable'. Grave and wise nods of agreement from other successful candidates abound. There are those, however, that will flinch as if suffering excruciating pain, mortally wounded on the battlefield, as they relive the horrors that have befallen them in previous attempts.

This book has been written with the intention of guiding MRCPCH (and DCH) candidates smoothly through the transition from fledgling to white swan (and just maybe a hawk or dove one day!). We have questioned past candidates over the last 10 years on the children they have seen in the exam and incorporated over 95% of them into this book in one form or another. We have provided 'stock' findings to the conditions and diseases encountered and added extras to enable the candidate to shine. It cannot take the place of, but can be used most efficiently in conjunction with, seeing patients and being examined under exam conditions.

We hope that you too may soon be a 'nodder' rather than the crestfallen.

Alan Cade
Donald Hodge

January 2000

Foreword

The authors of this book are specialist registrars who are not too old to have forgotten the traumas and stresses of the membership examination, although perhaps it can be argued that the memory of this particular life event never dims with age! The examination to gain membership of the Royal College of Paediatrics and Child Health is a major hurdle in one's professional training and the short cases are seen by many as the most testing component. Prospective examinees will find that this book not only provides a wide variety of clinical cases likely to be encountered during the examination but also gives practical advice regarding the examination technique itself.

Rather than simply presenting groups of short cases, the authors have produced a series of examination scenarios. For ease of reference, these have been arranged alphabetically in a dictionary format. The structure is based on how one might expect the short case examination to be conducted. Each 'case' is framed by a simple question followed by a specimen answer in which the main relevant points are highlighted in italics. There follows a series of notes pertinent to the question.

Examination success also marks the definitive start of the five year specialist training towards a consultant appointment and a book such as *Short Cases in Paediatrics* not only prepares the fledgling paediatrician for Membership but also provides a useful and instructive guide to the common, and not so common, conditions that are likely to be encountered in one's future career. In both the ward and clinic environment the paediatrician is, in fact, faced with a succession of 'short cases' and must develop the ability to recognize such conditions as the authors here describe. Thus, although books can never be a replacement for thorough clinical practice and experience, this volume should not only be seen as a means of passing the Membership exam but should also be viewed as a valuable aid in helping paediatricians develop their clinical skills.

Philip Holland
Consultant Paediatrician
Leeds General Infirmary

March 2000

Acknowledgements

Thanks are due to the following for their help:

Mr MD Stringer, Consultant Paediatric Surgeon, Clarendon Wing, Leeds General Infirmary, Leeds LS2 9NS, UK

Dr G Butler, Consultant Paediatric Endocrinologist, Clarendon Wing, Leeds General Infirmary, Leeds LS2 9NS, UK

Dr JWL Puntis, Consultant Paediatric Gastroenterologist, Clarendon Wing, Leeds General Infirmary, Leeds LS2 9NS, UK

Dr RJ Arthur, Consultant Paediatric Radiologist, Clarendon Wing, Leeds General Infirmary, Leeds LS2 9NS, UK

Dr PAJ Chetcuti, Consultant Respiratory Paediatrician, Clarendon Wing, Leeds General Infirmary, Leeds LS2 9NS, UK

Mr N George, Consultant Ophthalmologist, Clarendon Wing, Leeds General Infirmary, Leeds LS2 9NS, UK

Sister Gill Abel, Nutritional nurse specialist, Clarendon Wing, Leeds General Infirmary, Leeds LS2 9NS, UK

List of abbreviations used

ACTH adrenocorticotrophic hormone

AD autosomal dominant

AIDS acquired immunodeficiency syndrome

ALL acute lymphoblastic leukemia

ANA antinuclear antigen

ANF antinuclear factor

A-P diameter – anterior-posterior diameter

AR autosomal recessive

ASD atrial septal defect

ASOT anti-streptolysin O titre

A-V malformation arterio-venous malformation

BP blood pressure

BPD bronchopulmonary dysplasia

bpm beats per minute

CDH congenital dislocation of the hip

CGG cytosine, guanine, guanine

CK creatinine kinase

CMV cytomegalovirus

CNS central nervous system

CPK creatinine phosphokinase

CPR cardio-pulmonary resuscitation

CRP C-reactive protein

CSF cerebrospinal fluid

CT computerised tomography

CTG cytosine, thymidine, guanine

CVA cerebro-vascular accident

CXR chest X-ray

DCH diploma of child health

DDH developmental dysplasia of the hip

DEXA dual emission X-ray absorption

DIC disseminated intravascular coagulopathy

DMD Duchenne muscular dystrophy

DNA deoxyribonucleic acid

DVT deep vein thrombosis

EBV Ebstein Barr virus

ECG electrocardiogram

EEG electroencephalogram

EHBA extra-hepatic biliary atresia

EMG electromyelogram

ESR erythrocyte sedimentation rate

FBC full blood count

Fe iron

FSH follicular stimulating hormone

GP general practitioner

GN glomerulonephritis

Hb haemoglobin

HIV human immunodeficiency virus

HOCM hypertrophic obstructive cardiomyopathy

HSP Henoch–Schönlein purpura

IBD inflammatory bowel disease

ICP intracranial pressure

IDDM insulin dependent diabetes mellitus

IQ intelligence quotient

IRT immunoreactive trypsin

ITP idiopathic thrombocytopenic purpura

iv intravenous

IVC inferior vena cava

IVIG intravenous immunoglobulin

IVP intravenous pyelogram

JCA juvenile chronic arthritis

L left

LDL low density lipoprotein

LFT's liver function tests

LH luteinizing hormone

LMN lower motor neurone

LP lumbar puncture

MAC mid-arm circumference

MCV mean cell volume

MCP metacarpo-phalangeal

MD myotonic dystrophy

MG myasthenia gravis

MRCPCH Membership of the Royal College of Paediatrics and Child Health

MRI magnetic resonance imaging

NAI non-accidental injury

NSAID non-steroidal anti-inflammatory agents

OFC occipito-frontal circumference

PA pulmonary artery

PCD primary ciliary dyskinesia

PDA patent ductus arteriosus

PEF(R) peak expiratory flow (rate)

PKD polycystic kidney disease

PKU phenylketonuria

PV plasma vicosity

PWS Prader Willi syndrome

R right

RBC red blood cell

RF rheumatoid factor

RP retinitis pigmentosa

SLE systemic lupus erythematosis

SMA spinal muscular atrophy

TB tuberculosis

TOF tracheo-oesophageal atresia

TORCH taxoplasma, rubella, cytomegalovirus herpes

U&E's urea and electrolytes

UK United Kingdom

URTI upper respiratory tract infection

USA United States of America

USS ultrasound scan

VLCFA very long chain fatty acids

VLDL very low density lipoprotein

VP ventriculo-peritoneal

VSD ventricular septal defect

WCC white cell count

Introduction

By the time you reach the clinical section of the part 2 MRCPCH, your knowledge base will be enormous (hopefully!) and may never be as good again! However, listing 14 causes for an ingrowing toenail 'off-pat' sadly will not be enough to get you through this section of the examination. What is required now is for you to put the paediatric textbooks back on the shelf (apart from this one!), next to the dusty Gray's Anatomy and actually see some pathology 'hands on'.

Those candidates who have struggled through part 1 and the written section of part 2 are often those that shine in the clinical sections. This person is often the last to come forward offering to examine patients in front of others; the quiet unassuming type, but performs superbly when given the opportunity. Thoroughness, yet speed, is required together with anticipation about the thought processes of the examiners. These are not easy skills to learn, but practise on patients and each other is far more productive than reading the books.

The art of the short case is to be able to examine an organ system or part of the human anatomy as if it were second nature. If your thoughts are about what more you need to do to complete the pertinent examination properly rather than interpretation of your positive (and negative) findings to formulate a (differential) diagnosis, then you will flounder. 'Cases' brought forward for this part of the examination are usually well children with stable pathologies. Although the possibilities are limitless, certain diseases lend themselves very well to this part of the exam and in reality the same cases are seen time and time again.

The exam generally is run extremely efficiently and fairly, although all of us can recount horror stories of the torture we endured at the hands of particular examiners. It is striking how little the exam has changed over the last decade apart perhaps from the retirement of some very well known 'hawks'. Sadly, others have come through the ranks and may be there to test your resilience!

The short cases format

You have 30 minutes for the short cases during which time you will have 2 examiners, each having 15 minutes to assess your abilities. Invariably you will have just completed your long case and you must push thoughts of this to the back of your mind (you will have plenty of opportunity to reminisce about your exam on the way home!). There is no truth in the belief that some examiners fail more than others and so recognising a particular 'ungenerous' examiner on the opposite side of bed must not put you off. Their fellow examiners are there to ensure fair play. This person may disappear at times, however, and again this should not distract you from the job in hand.

Invariably, the examination room is noisy and appears chaotic. Fellow examinees may be heard being put through their paces only yards away. Do not pay them any attention. You may well see the same patient they are seeing and if you have heard them make a diagnosis you may bias your subsequent examination and answers. They may be right but they may also be wrong!

Inevitably as soon as the letter arrives telling the candidate where they will be going to do the clinical section of the Part 2, there is a degree of trying to anticipate what the likely cases will be. There is little to be gained by doing this and it may in fact be counter-productive. If, for example, your exam is at a tertiary referral centre for metabolic disorders, you may expect any child with hepatomegaly to have a glycogen storage disorder. You may choose to ignore the central sternotomy scar and central cyanosis, together with hepatomegaly, consistent with complex congenital heart disease and right-sided heart failure. We would therefore advise against such guesswork as it may only cloud your better judgement.

Similarly trying to anticipate who your likely examiners are going to be can be unhelpful. Certain institutions may be well known for their 'hawkish' examiners but commonly they are either not examining at all or they are the external examiner for another centre. If you are sufficiently well prepared, you should not care who you will meet at the opposite side of the patient scrutinising your every word and action.

Equipment – to take or not to take, that is the question!

There is no right or wrong answer to this. The examination centres should provide everything you need to conduct the requested examinations. Some people do, however, prefer to use their own and this should be encouraged for the sake of familiarity and availability. If you choose to amass your own 'box of tricks' make sure that you have used it before in practice sessions. In the heat of the moment it is very easy to leave some or all of your equipment behind with the last patient – this causes big problems for you and the examination team. **If you take your own, keep it with you.** Below is a suggested list of items for inclusion:

- Paper for drawing on
- Several pencils/crayons (for you to draw and the child to imitate if necessary)
- Six different coloured building blocks
- An ophthalmoscope
- Cotton wool ball
- Pen torch
- Toy car
- Smarties, raisins, cake decorations
- Tape measure/ruler
- Picture book

Examination

Listen carefully to what the examiner asks you to do. If you are unsure, then clarify the situation but do not repeat their instructions just for the sake of it.

Introduce yourself to the patient and parent. Cast a general eye over the patient and their surroundings for clues to the diagnosis. Even if not directly relevant to the examination of the system or organ you are looking at, it is worthwhile commenting on obvious features of importance, e.g. the child is in a wheelchair, there are no spontaneous movements of his lower limbs, he is wearing bilateral hearing aids. Once a general inspection is completed, ask the child or guardian if they (the child) have any pain or tenderness anywhere. Take control of the examination, explaining exactly what it is you're going to do to the child. Do not ask the child '*Is it alright if I . . .?*'. If the child says no, you then have a problem!

Full exposure without losing modesty, if appropriate, is essential and you may have to help the child take their clothes off. Once again, stand back and note any general observations, e.g. the presence of scars, surgical lines, enterostomies, dyspnoea. Having practised your examination routine (see examination techniques) for each system so many times before you should now be able to run through this without thought, following any instructions the examiner gives. Your attention and thought should be on piecing together the information gathered to come up with a (differential) diagnosis. Once done, help the child to get dressed and thank them for allowing you to examine them. **Never hurt the patient.**

Never make up signs – it is suicidal! If you cannot detect any abnormality then say so. You could be examining a normal child (perhaps the examiner's own child brought in for the exam because of a shortage of suitable patients – they will not appreciate you telling them their child is dysmorphic, if they are not!).

Presentation

Examiners will differ in how the examination and presentation should be undertaken. Some may want you to talk through what you are doing and finding as you go along, whilst others will want a résumé of your findings at the end. Either way, by the time you have finished your examination, you should already have a very good idea about the likely diagnosis. If the latter approach is adopted, and you are sure, then start your presentation by saying '*Steven has Poland syndrome . . .*'. Back this up by listing the positive findings you have demonstrated (and other findings that you would want to look for if you had the opportunity). If you are unsure about the specific diagnosis, then give a differential. If you are completely clueless then simply present your findings and hope they do not ask you for the answer (they may not know it either!). Very often, however, the examiner will push you to commit yourself to making a diagnosis. Think logically before you speak, e.g. do not say that a girl has Duchenne muscular dystrophy. If you really haven't got a clue then admit that you are baffled.

You must articulate your presentation clearly and in an appropriate order. Do it as if you were phoning your consultant for advice about a patient you have seen on the ward. Confidence, both in examination technique and presentation skills, is half the battle. This comes to some more easily than others, but practise, practise, practise before the examination day will work wonders.

Do not be dogmatic, but at the same time do not be hesitant. *'This child has splenomegaly of 3 cm below the left costal margin'* sounds much more professional than *'I think this child may have 1 or 2 finger-breadths of splenomegaly, but I cannot feel a notch so it may be something else'*. **Never argue with the examiner**, but do not agree with everything they say. Instead discuss logically why you think what you do and state why you do not agree with their point of view.

Keep your cool! You may well make mistakes and miss something that the examiner will kindly point out to you! It is said that if you miss a scar you will fail regardless, but if you have been brilliant otherwise, you may get away with it. Do not get phased – it really isn't over 'until the fat lady sings' and you must stay composed throughout, even if things are going badly. Do not show hostility towards the examiner even if you feel they are not being very generous. **Do not expect positive or negative feedback.** However, if the former is given do not become complacent and if the latter is proffered, do not crumple!

Examination techniques

Cardiovascular examination

The cardiovascular examination remains one of the most common short cases. This is probably due to the simple fact that the clinical features are long-standing and specific and more importantly, there are a large number of well children walking around with good clinical signs. Given these facts it is imperative that a candidate performs well and is able to elicit all the clinical signs. In order to do this, it is important to have a basic understanding of human anatomy and physiology. Cardiovascular examination is not difficult and most of the mistakes made are due to accidental omission of critically important parts of the examination such as measuring the blood pressure or assessing the femoral pulses. The examination technique outlined below should be regarded as a skeleton framework, which to us is logical and not too difficult to remember even under the most stressful conditions.

The dilemma of whether to talk to the examiner throughout your examination or to simply present the findings after a period of silent examination (hoping that the examiner can tell what you have been doing) is commonly encountered. We do not feel that there is a right answer to this but suggest that a mixture of the two is best. Specifically, we would recommend talking your way through the 'peripheral cardio-vascular examination' so the examiner knows what you have been doing. This also helps to keep the examiner awake as often they have had a long day. Before examining the precordium let the examiner know that you will present your findings at the end. By doing this, the examiner will know why you have suddenly 'shut up' and will be able to concentrate on your expert examination technique.

1. Introduce yourself to both parent and child
2. During the introduction, you should be making a 'mental survey' of the child looking for any clues
   - Is the child cyanosed?
   - Is the child breathless?
   - Is the child's nutrition good?
   - Does the child have any obvious syndrome or dysmorphic features?
     - Down's, William's, Marfan's, Turner's, Alagille's
3. Expose the child's chest and place in a comfortable position (in bed, on parent's knee)
4. Examination of hands
   - Clubbing
     - look at all fingers
     - be seen to look at the nail angle against the horizon
     - note: clubbing first appears in the thumbs
   - Look at all nails (infective endocarditis)
   - Splinter haemorrhages
   - Peripheral cyanosis

- comment if present although important to say it may be environmental
5. Assessment of pulse – child < 3 years old – brachial pulse; child > 3 years old – radial pulse
   - Rate – feel for 15 seconds and multiply by 4 – **never guess**
   - Rhythm – sinus, irregular?
   - Character – collapsing, plateau pulse, full?
   - Volume
   - Femoral pulses – ask to assess at this stage
     - radial-femoral delay only clinically detectable in children > 12 years old with coarctation
6. Face
   - Conjunctivae – pallor
   - Sclerae – jaundice
   - Tongue – central cyanosis (definition: > 5 g/dl of deoxygenated haemoglobin)
   - Teeth – comment on any dental caries
7. JVP
   - Consider assessing in the neck of a child > 12 years old. Difficult before this age
8. Inspection of the chest – must expose chest fully
   - Respiratory rate – count for 15 seconds and times by 4 – **never guess**
   - Shape of chest wall – asymmetry
   - Scars
     - Left lateral thoracotomy
       - coarctation repair
       - left Blalock–Taussig shunt
       - PDA ligation
       - PA banding
     - Right lateral thoracotomy
       - right Blalock–Taussig shunt
       - tracheo-oesophageal fistula repair
     - Sub-mammary incision
       - ASD repair (approach used in girl's)
     - Central sternotomy
       - reconstructive surgery (ASD, VSD, Fallot's)
       - valvular surgery
       - any procedure that requires the patient to be on cardiopulmonary bypass
9. Palpation
   - Apex beat – feel for the most lateral and inferior pulsation ? with right hand (beware dextrocardia). Once found palpate the anterior sternum for the angle of Louis (2nd intercostal space) and count down to meet your right hand. Normal position in children 4th–5th intercostal space in the midclavicular space)

- Thrills – palpable murmur. Murmur > grade 4/6 to have a thrill
  - Grade 1 – very soft
  - Grade 2 – soft
  - Grade 3 – moderate
  - Grade 4 – loud
  - Grade 5 – very loud
  - Grade 6 – very loud (no stethoscope needed)
- Heaves – left parasternal heave – right ventricular hypertrophy
- Palpable S_2 – pulmonary areas – pulmonary hypertension

10. Auscultation

In children it is difficult to differentiate the first and second heart sound due to the fast heart rate. Therefore, place your left hand on the child's right brachial pulse in order to time the cardiac cycle.

- S_1
  - mitral and tricuspid valve shutting
  - start of systole (contraction)
  - synchronous with pulse
- S_2
  - aortic and pulmonary valve shutting
  - start of diastole (relaxation)

Listen to all 4 valve areas (Figure 1) with the diaphragm and only the mitral and tricuspid areas with the bell. If a murmur is heard – loudest area, intensity, timing in cardiac cycle, radiation (e.g. into neck). Do not listen in the neck for a murmur if you haven't heard one on the precordium. Sit child forward and listen between the scapulae.

11. Lung fields
- Sit child forward and listen to both lung bases for evidence of pulmonary oedema (left heart failure)
- Feel for sacral oedema (right heart failure)

12. Abdomen – ask the examiner if you can palpate the abdomen for evidence of hepatomegaly (heart failure) and splenomegaly (bacterial endocarditis)

13. Peripheral pulses – tell the examiner that you would like to conclude your examination by making a full assessment of all the peripheral pulses

14. Blood pressure
- Use a cuff that covers at least 2/3 of the upper arm
- Always use right arm (pre-ductal)
- Have cuff at same level as heart
- Korotkoff sounds
  - 1st phase – sounds appear (systolic pressure)
  - 4th phase – sounds become muffled
  - 5th phase – sounds disappear (diastolic pressure)

Respiratory examination

This is a common short case and one that examiners expect to be performed well. The text below outlines a skeleton on which to base the examination.

1. Introduce yourself to both parent and child
2. During the introduction you should be making a 'mental survey' of the child looking for any clues
   - Is the child cyanosed?
   - Nutritional status?
   - Ex-premature baby? – scaphocephaly, VP shunt, glasses?
   - Cushingoid?
   - Is the child in respiratory distress? – intercostal/subcostal recession, tracheal tug, respiratory rate, grunting (breathing against a partially closed glottis)
   - Any stridor, audible wheeze, cough?
   - Normal chest movement?
   - Any clues around the bed – nebuliser, PEF meter, Creon, sputum pot, oxygen, saturation monitor
3. Expose the child's chest and place in a comfortable position (in bed, on parent's knee)
4. Examination of hands
   - Clubbing
     - look at all fingers
     - be seen to look at the nail angle against the horizon
   - Peripheral cyanosis
     - Comment if present although important to say it may be environmental
5. Assessment of pulse – Child < 3 years old – brachial pulse; child > 3 years old – radial pulse
   - Rate – feel for 15 seconds and multiply by 4 – **never guess**
6. Face
   - Eyes – anaemia (look at conjuctivae)
   - Tongue – cyanosis (look under tongue for central cyanosis)
7. Ask the child to perform a 'big cough' for you – a fruity, productive sounding cough would make a diagnosis of cystic fibrosis more likely
8. Examination of chest

Inspection of chest
- Respiratory rate – count for 15 seconds and multiply by 4 – **never guess**
- Scars – look at all of the chest (front and back)
- Respiratory pattern – normal, respiratory distress?
- Chest shape
  - pectus excavatum
  - pectus carinatum

- Harrison's sulci
- scoliosis
- hyperinflation ($\uparrow$A–P diameter)

Palpation of chest

In order to look slick we would recommend performing palpation, percussion and auscultation on the front of the chest and then sitting the child forward and performing the same on the back.

- Trachea
  - feel if the trachea is central (only do this in children > 3 years old as younger children will get upset)
- Apex beat
  - feel for the most inferior and lateral pulsation
  - isolate the position from the 2nd intercostal space (angle of Louis)
- Expansion – appropriate in children over 5 years of age
  - ask child to take a big breath in and out; this will give an idea of expansion
  - place the fingers of both hands on the lateral chest wall with the thumbs meeting in the midline
  - ask the child to take a big breath in and look at the movement of the thumbs (it is very difficult to look as if you are not fiddling the result)
- Tactile vocal fremitus – appropriate in children over 5 years of age
  - Place the ulnar side of your hand on the upper anterior chest wall
  - ask the child to say '99'
  - compare both sides
    - $\uparrow$ vibration – consolidation
    - $\downarrow$ vibration – pneumothorax
    - Absent/ $\downarrow$ vibration – pleural effusion

Percussion of chest

This should be performed on the front of the chest with the child sitting forward and the same performed on the back. It should not be performed on children < 2–3 years old as they will be scared.

- Tell the child that you are going to make their chest sound like a drum
- Important to have finger that is being percussed parallel to the ribs to avoid transmission of sound from more than one rib space
- Percuss the clavicles and the axilla on both sides and then 3 sites on both sides of the chest. Percuss 3 areas on each side of the back
- It is important to compare sides – percuss one area on the left side of the chest and then percuss the same area on the right
- Perform only two taps in each area

Percussion note	Diagnosis
Resonant	Normal
Hyperresonant	Pneumothorax
Dull	Consolidation
Stony dull	Pleural fluid

Auscultation of the chest

The chest should be listened to with the diaphragm of the stethoscope in the same areas that were percussed.

- Normal breath sounds – vesicular
- Pleural effusion – absent breath sounds
- Collapse – decreased vesicular
- Consolidation – bronchial breathing
  - inspiratory and expiratory sounds are blowing in nature
  - expiration as long and loud as inspiration
  - pause between inspiration and expiration
- Added sounds – wheeze, crackles, pleural rub

9. Ask the child to lean forward and perform expansion, percussion and auscultation on his back
10. ENT examination – tell the examiner that you would like to make a full examination of the child's ears, nose and throat, including a full assessment of lymphadenopathy
11. PEFR – tell the examiner that to conclude your examination you would like to assess the child's peak flow (in children over 5 years of age)

Abdominal examination

The abdominal examination is probably the easiest of all the systems to examine. We would recommend talking to the examiner throughout 'the peripheral abdominal examination' (to keep the examiner awake) and explaining that you will examine the abdomen and present your findings at the end.

1. Introduce yourself to parents and child
2. During the introduction you should be making a 'mental survey' of the child looking for any clues, e.g. race (thalassaemia, sickle cell disease), jaundice, bruising, dysmorphic features
3. Position the child sitting up on the bed
4. Examination of the hands
   - Clubbing
     - examine the nailbed against the horizon
     - examine both hands
   - Nails
     - leuconychia
     - koilonychia

- Palmar erythema
  - liver disease
5. Face
  - Eyes
    - jaundice
    - anaemia
  - Mouth
    - ulceration (IBD, Behçet's)
    - pigmentation (Peutz-Jeghers syndrome)
  - Lips
    - swollen lips (Crohn's disease)
  - Spider naevi
    - > 3 in the area drained by the superior vena cava is significant
6. Lie child down flat on the bed or guardian's lap, with their abdomen exposed. Do not expose genitalia
7. Inspection of abdomen
  - Scars (be sure to look in renal angles)
  - Distention
  - Masses
  - Striae
  - Prominent abdominal veins
  - Gastrostomy, ileostomy, colostomy, vesicostomy
8. Palpation of abdomen
  - **Be sure to ask child if abdomen is painful prior to starting**
  - Lightly palpate the entire abdomen with the palm of right hand
  - Be sure to watch the child's face throughout and be seen to be doing so
  - Deeply palpate the entire abdomen. Continue to look at child's face

Next move on to identification of each abdominal organ in turn. Palpate each organ and percuss it before moving onto the next organ.

Liver
Palpation – Start in the right iliac fossa using your right hand. Ask child to breathe in and co-ordinate palpation with inspiration. Describe the texture and firmness of the liver.

Percussion – Start above the liver in the chest and percuss down in the mid-clavicular line (easier to differentiate resonant → dull).

(Notes: Liver – smooth edge, moves with respiration, cannot get above it, dull to percussion.)

Spleen
Palpation – Start in the right iliac fossa and palpate upwards towards the upper left quadrant. Ask child to breathe in and co-ordinate palpation with inspiration. Roll child onto right side and feel under the left costal margin to see if you can tip a spleen.

Percussion – Start in the right iliac fossa and percuss up towards the left upper quadrant.

(Notes: Spleen – moves with respiration, cannot get above it, dull to percussion, notch on medial surface.)

Kidney

Palpation – Ballot each kidney in turn. Keep right hand on abdomen and use left hand underneath.

Percussion – Percuss over both kidneys.

(Notes: Kidney – moves with respiration, can get above them, ballottable, resonant to percussion.)

9. Auscultation of abdomen
   • Listen to abdomen for presence of bowel sounds
   • Listen over both kidneys for bruit
10. Anus, genitalia, hernial orifices
   • Tell the examiner that you would like to examine the anus, perineum, genitalia and hernial orifices. In reality you would never be asked to do this but you must offer to do so.

Neurological examination

Many candidates often fear performing a neurological examination. The reasoning behind this probably reflects a universal lack of practice. There is nothing particularly difficult about the examination but the trick is making it look like you have done it many times before. The following presents a logical way of examining the upper limb, lower limb, cranial nerves, gait, cerebellar examination and finally developmental assessment, all of which are common short cases.

Upper limb examination

The following outline presents a skeleton from which to base all examinations of the upper limbs. It should, of course, be tailored to the age of the child. We suggest talking to the examiner throughout. It is important to know dermatomes and nerve roots for reflexes – they're not that difficult to remember!

1. Introduce yourself to both parent and child
2. During the introduction you should be making a 'mental survey' of the child looking for any clues, e.g. wheelchair, orthoses, helmet, dysmorphic features

3. Ask child/parent to expose chest and both arms
4. Inspection of arms and chest
   • Posture
     • Erb's palsy – C5, 6
     • Klumpke palsy – C8, T1
   • Contractures
   • Muscle bulk
   • Muscle wasting
   • Involuntary movements
   • Fasciculation
   • Scars

   (Remember to compare both arms)

5. Tone
   • Hold onto hand and passively move arm in unexpected, irregular way
   • Passive pronation/supination of both forearms
   • Test both arms
6. Power – important to know the grading of power and to compare both sides. Grade each muscle group out of 5 as below:
   • Grade 0 – no movement
   • Grade 1 – flicker of contraction
   • Grade 2 – movement if gravity removed
   • Grade 3 – movement against gravity but not resistance
   • Grade 4 – movement against resistance
   • Grade 5 – normal power

   Shoulder abduction – C5
   'Put your arms out by your side as if you were a bird. Push your arms away from your body. Don't let me stop you.'

   Shoulder adduction – C5, 6, 7 and 8
   'Put your arms out by your side as if you were a bird. Pull your arms into your body. Don't let me stop you.'

   Elbow flexion – C5, 6
   'Bend your arms and hold them in front of you. Pull me towards you.'

   Elbow extension – C7, 8
   'Bend your arms and hold them in front of you. Push me away.'

   Hand – C8, T1
   'Squeeze my fingers'
   – C8, T1
   'Spread your fingers wide. Don't let me squeeze them together.'

7. Reflexes – compare both sides
   • Biceps – C5, 6
   • Triceps – C7, 8
   • Brachioradialis – C5, 6

8. Co-ordination
   - Finger-nose touching (dysmetria) – *'Touch your nose then touch my finger.'* Must move your finger to different sites.
   - Hand tapping (dysdiadochokinesia) – *'Tap one hand on the back of the other. Alternate tapping with the palm and the back of the hand.'* (Most children will need to have this demonstrated to them.)
9. Sensation – very difficult to perform in children. Important to have a rough idea about dermatomes (see below). Test light touch, vibration. (Pain sensation not usually expected to be tested in children.)
   - C4 – tip of shoulder
   - C5 – upper outer border of arm
   - C6 – lateral lower arm (radial border)
   - C7 – radial surface of middle finger
   - C8 – ulnar border of hand
   - T1 – lower arm, medial surface
   - T2 – upper arm, medial surface
   - T3 – axilla

   - Spinothalamic pathway
     - Pain and temperature sensation
     - Fibres enter the spinal cord, cross the midline and pass up the spinothalamic tracts

   - Posterior columns
     - Proprioception, fine touch and vibration sensation
     - Fibres ascend in the posterior column to the medulla and then cross the midline
10. Function – assess the child drawing/scribbling/writing/picking up small objects

Lower limb examination

This is a more common short case than the upper limb. This is because it is easier to examine, the signs are easily reproducible and there are more children with physical signs available to come to examinations. Examination of the child's gait is a very important part of the examination and is dealt with as a separate short case later.

1. Introduce yourself to both parent and child
2. During the introduction you should be making 'a mental survey' of the child, looking for any clues, e.g. wheelchair, orthoses, helmet, splints, dysmorphic features.
3. Ask the child to strip to underpants only (important to look at back)
4. Assess gait (see below)

5. Inspection – spine and legs. Position child lying on bed
   - Posture
   - Contractions
   - Muscle bulk
   - Muscle wasting
   - Muscle pseudohypertrophy/hypertrophy
   - Involuntary movements
   - Fasciculation
   - Scars
6. Tone – roll legs from side to side (irregular, unpredictable movements)
7. Power – see grading of power above. Compare both sides

   Hip flexion – L1, 2, 3
   'Lift your leg straight off the bed, don't let me stop you.'

   Hip extension – L5, S1
   'Press your leg onto the bed, don't let me lift your leg up.'

   Knee flexion – L3, 4
   'Bend knee to 90°. Kick me away, don't let me stop you.'

   Knee extension – S1
   'Bend knee to 90°. Pull your knee towards your bottom, don't let me stop you.'

   Ankle flexion – S1, 2
   Place hand on sole of foot *'Push my hand away (like a car accelerator), don't let me stop you.'*

   Ankle extension – L4
   Place hand on dorsum of foot. *'Pull your toes up towards you, don't let me stop you.'*

8. Reflexes – test both sides
   - Knee reflex – L3, 4
   - Ankle reflex – S1, 2
   - Plantar reflex – abnormal result: up-going big toe and splaying of toes (stroke finger up lateral aspect of sole of foot and medially across ball of foot). The plantar is normally up-going in infants until they begin to walk
9. Co-ordination – test both sides
   - Ask the child to run the heel of one foot down the shin of the other (heel-shin test).
10. Sensation – very difficult to perform in children. Important to have a rough idea about dermatomes (see below). Test light touch, vibration. (Pain sensation not usually expected to be tested in children.)
    - L1 – upper outer thigh
    - L2 – middle anterior thigh
    - L3 – anterior knee

- L4 – medial calf
- L5 – lateral calf
- S1 – sole of foot
- S2 – strip up posterior calf and thigh

11. Clonus – test both ankles (dorsiflex foot rapidly); > 3 beats of ankle clonus is abnormal

Gait

Examination of gait is generally performed poorly. The examination itself is not difficult to do and therefore the poor performance probably reflects a lack of practice. A method on which to base the examination is outlined below.

1. Introduce yourself to both parent and child
2. During the introduction you should be making a 'mental survey' of the child, looking for any clues, e.g. wheelchair, orthoses, helmet, splints, abnormal posture, abnormal movements, dysmorphic features
3. Strip child down to underwear only (if appropriate)
4. Examination of back – ? scars
5. Inspection of legs
   - Pain
   - Hypertrophy/wasting
   - Shortening
   - Scars
6. Ask the child to walk normally across room
   - Does heel/forefoot touch ground first?
   - Is the foot position in valgus/varus?
   - Movement of knee
   - Noise of walking (Does foot slap onto floor?)
   - Obvious limp
   - Arm position
   - Position during walking
   - Any abnormal movements
7. Ask child to heel–toe walk
   - Only reliable in children > 3 years old
   - Tests cerebellar pathways
8. Ask child to walk on outsides of feet (Fog's test)
   - Exacerbates signs of a subtle hemiplegia
9. Ask child to run
   - Exacerbates signs of a subtle hemiplegia
10. Squat–stand
    - Ask child to stand from squatting
    - Assesses for proximal myopathy
11. Trendelenberg's sign
    - Ask the patient to stand in front of you facing away

- Ask the patient to lift one foot off the ground
  - normal – pelvis lifts on the side of the lifted leg
  - abnormal – sagging pelvis on the side of lifted leg
12. Gower's sign
  - Ask the child to stand from lying **supine**
  - Tests for proximal weakness
  (A normal child will simply sit up from lying and then stand. A child with DMD will have to roll over onto their front and then climb up their legs.)

13. Examine the child's shoes for evidence of abnormal wearing

Cranial nerves

It is essential to be able to perform a cranial nerve examination. The examination is not difficult but it is easy to appear as if you have never done it before. A knowledge of the cranial nerves on its own will not suffice and it is important to practise the examination. Below is an outline of each cranial nerve in detail and a skeleton on which to base the examination.

I Olfactory nerve

Smell
Examination: test each nostril separately.

II Optic nerve

Visual acuity
Examination: important to test visual acuity first to confirm that the child can see.

- Child 2–3 years old – assess with a toy
- Child age 3 – stycar matching letters
- Child > 5 years – formally with Snellen chart

Visual fields
Examination: test by confrontation perimetry. This is difficult to perform in younger children. Ask older children to sit opposite you and cover their right eye with their right hand and look at your nose with their left eye. You should cover the opposite eye on yourself. Ask the child when they can see your fingers moving. Test both eyes. (It is important that you know the visual pathway so you can interpret results.)

Fundoscopy
Examination: should be performed in all examinations. In reality, the examiners will not ask you to do this unless there is pathology to be seen.

Common fundoscopy short cases: optic atrophy, papilloedema, retinitis pigmentosa, cherry red spot, coloboma, aniridia, cataract.

III Oculomotor nerve

Efferent fibres to superior, inferior and medial recti, inferior oblique, levator palpebral superioris muscles. Parasympathetic supply to eye.

3rd nerve palsy
- Unilateral ptosis
- Eye – down and out
- Fixed, dilated pupil

Examination: see below.

IV Trochlear nerve

Supplies superior oblique muscle.

4th nerve palsy
- Diplopia on looking down and away from the affected side

Examination: see below.

V Trigeminal nerve

Motor
- Muscles of mastication

Examination: *'Open your mouth, don't let me close it.'* Deviation to the side of weakness. Clench teeth tight together – feel muscle mass.

Sensory
- Ophthalmic, maxillary, mandibular divisions. Corneal sensation.

Examination: test each division on each side of the face. Corneal sensation – this should never be tested in the conscious child.

VI Abducens nerve

Supplies lateral rectus muscle.

6th nerve palsy
- Convergent squint
- Failure of abduction beyond midline on affected side

Examination: ask the child to fix and follow on an object. Observe eye movements throughout all quadrants.

VII Facial nerve

Motor
- Muscles of facial expression

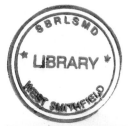

Sensory
• Taste – anterior 2/3 of tongue

LMN lesion
• Weakness ipsilateral

UMN lesion
• Weakness contralateral (frontalis spared)

Examination: ask the child to screw-up eyes, raise eyebrows, blow out cheeks, show teeth.

VIII Vestibulocochlear

Cochlear division
• Hearing

Vestibular division
• Balance and posture

Examination: candidates should be able to perform Rinne's/Weber's test, describe how to perform a hearing distraction test, interpret results of caloric testing.

Caloric testing
Assesses function of the labyrinth. Look at the direction of nystagmus when ice-cold water and then warm water is run against the tympanic membrane. Normal – eyes look away from ice-cold water and towards warm water, e.g.

• cold water in left ear – eyes to right
• warm water in left ear – eyes to left
• cold water in right ear – eyes to left
• warm water in right ear – eyes to right

Hearing distraction test
This test requires two examiners, parent and child. The parent sits with the child on their knee. The distracter kneels in front of the child with a toy and obtains the child's attention with care not to make a sound. The examiner stands behind the child and signals to the distracter to remove the toy. The examiner then makes a sound 1 meter behind the child with care not to enter the child's visual field. The response of the child to the noise is recorded. The test is repeated for the other ear. Ideally, the test is done in a sound-proof room with overhead lighting (so shadows do not distract the child).

Weber's test
Place a vibrating tuning fork in the middle of the child's forehead. Ask the child which ear he/she hears the noise in loudest.

• Normal – L = R
• Conductive deafness – Loudest in affected ear
• Sensorineural deafness – Loudest on normal side

Rinne's test
Place the tuning fork next to the ear. Ask the child whether they can hear it. Next, place the tuning fork on the mastoid process. Ask the child which is louder.

- Conductive deafness – bone loudest (bone conduction better than air conduction)
- Sensorineural deafness – air loudest (air conduction better than bone conduction)

IX Glossopharyngeal

Motor
- Stylopharyngeus muscle

Sensory
- Taste – posterior 1/3 tongue
- Sensation – tonsillar fossa and pharynx

Examination: see below.

X Vagus nerve

Motor
- Pharynx and larynx

Sensory
- Larynx

Examination: IX and X nerve tested together. *'Open your mouth, say aah.'* Look at palatal movement. Gag reflex – sensory (IX nerve), motor (X nerve).

XI Accessory nerve

Motor
- Trapezius and sternomastoid

Examination: ask child to shrug shoulders. Ask child to turn head to the right, place your hand on the left side of their face and ask child to push against your hand. Test the opposite direction.

XII Hypoglossal nerve

Motor
- Tongue

Examination: ask child to stick out tongue. Inspect for fasciculation (fasciculation – LMN lesion) and deviation (tongue deviates to side of lesion).

Cerebellum examination

1. Introduce yourself to parents and child
2. During the introduction, you should be making a 'mental survey' of the child, looking for any clues. Ask the child some questions.
   - Any abnormal movements?
   - Any abnormality in speech?
   - Any nystagmus?
3. Speech
   - Ask the child some questions (stuttering dysarthria)
4. Eyes
   - Look for evidence of horizontal nystagmus
   - Ask the child to fix on an object and move it to the extremes of lateral vision
5. Upper limbs

   Intention tremor
   - Ask the child to hold their hands out in front
   - Ask them to pick up a small object with either hand and look for evidence of a tremor

   Dysmetria
   - Ask the child to cover one eye with one hand and with the other hand (index finger) touch their nose and then touch your finger
   - Repeat this many times varying the position of your finger both in direction and in distance from the child
   - Repeat this with the other eye and finger

   Dysdiadokinesia
   - Ask the child to hold their right hand still and pat it with the left hand; Ask the child to do this as quickly as possible
   - Ask the child to alternate tapping the right hand with the palm and the back of the left hand as quickly as possible
   - Test both hands

   Piano playing
   - Ask the child to pretend to play an imaginary keyboard

6. Lower limbs

   Heel–shin test
   - With the child lying on the bed ask the child to lift the right foot off the bed and run the heel down the shin of the left leg
   - Do the same with the opposite leg

   Toe-tapping
   - Ask the child to tap your hand with the sole of the right foot as quickly as possible
   - Do the same with the other foot

Gait
- Ask the child to walk normally and then walk heel–toe
- Look for a broad-based ataxic gait

Developmental assessment

This is a very common short case. Despite this fact it is frequently poorly performed. The examination itself is not difficult but it is very difficult to look slick. It is important to remember that the assessment is really an exercise in observation and description rather than a 'hands-on' physical examination. It is essential to be familiar with key developmental milestones for children aged 3 months to 5 years old. These are listed in Table 1. A knowledge of primitive reflexes is also essential and the most common of these are described.

Table 1   Developmental milestones from 6 months to 5 years

Development	Gross	Fine motor and vision	Hearing and speech	Social
6 months	Sits ± support	Palmar grasp, transfers	Laughs, vocalises, responds to own name	Hand and foot regard, mouths objects
9 months	Crawls	Pincer grasp	Polysyllabic babbling	Plays 'peek-a-boo'
12 months	Pulls to stand, cruises	Points to objects, casts, holds 2 objects	Turns to sound of name, understands several words, 'mama', 'dada'	Drinks from a cup, waves, plays 'pat-a-cake'
18 months	Walks unaided, climbs onto a chair ± stairs	Scribbles, turns pages, builds a 3-block tower	Obeys simple instructions, 3 or more words, jabbers	Holds a spoon, takes off shoes and socks
2½ years	Climbs and descends stairs, kicks a ball, jumps	8-block tower, draws lines	Plurals, knows own name	Plays alone, dresses, dry by day
3 years	Runs, stands on 1 foot briefly, rides tricycle	Draws circle, threads beads	Sentences, knows age	Uses knife and fork, toilets alone
4 years	Hops, heel-to-toe, climbs ladders	Draws cross, square and basic man	Counts to 10, knows name, age, address and colours	Shares toys, brushes teeth
5 years	Catches a ball	Draws triangle, detailed man	Clear speech	Comforts others, group play

One approach to the assessment is outlined below. Given the age of children commonly used for this part of the examination, things can be rather unpredictable. Stand back at the start of the examination and observe the child. More than for any other short case it is important that you talk as you go along, explaining your actions if necessary. For example, do not be afraid to ask the parent whether the child has started rolling over yet or saying any recognisable words. You might get some clues from them if, for example, the child has just had their MMR vaccination or hearing assessment.

If asked at the end to give a developmental age for the child – **be careful**! Do not forget that the child may not perform to the best of their abilities in the exam (as may be the case for yourself!!) because of the environment. Parents may get upset if they have a normally developing child and you inform the examiner that the child's developmental age is less than their chronological age. If unsure then err on the side of caution and never be too specific. Saying a child's developmental age is 9–12 months is far safer than saying 10 months and you will not offend the parent if the child is 11 months old.

The developmental assessment is divided into 4 areas, all of which must be examined:

- Gross motor
- Fine motor and vision
- Hearing and speech
- Social skills.

Look at the child and try to guess in your mind how old the child is. For each of the above it is important to pitch the examination at an appropriate level. For example, if the child is running around the room when you walk in, do not lie them down and pull to sitting to look at head lag as the child has already demonstrated good head control. A good approach is to try to elicit developmental milestones that you would expect in a child age 3 months younger than you think the child is and progress forward trying to elicit more advanced milestones. Once you have elicited (or asked about) the most advanced milestone, proceed onto the next group. At the end of the exam present your findings to the examiners using the above 4 groups as headings.

1. Introduce yourself to child and parents
2. Perform a visual survey – dysmorphic features, ex-premature, posture, aids, contractures, asymmetry, e.g. hemiplegia
3. Gross motor
   - Start examination at appropriate level.

   Routine in baby
   - Lie child supine – posture?
   - Hold both arms and pull the child to sitting – head control?
   - Hold child in sitting position – sit unsupported?
   - Hold child in standing position – weight bear on legs?

- Ventral suspension – hold the child prone with your hand under the child's thorax. Hold child 1 foot above bed – head, trunk position?
- Prone – lower child onto bed and lie in prone position with arms out in front – head, trunk position?

- In the older child observe gait, kicking object, catching etc.

Primitive reflexes

It is important to assess primitive reflexes in infants. Persistence beyond the time period below is abnormal.

Rooting reflex

If the upper lip is stroked the baby will turn their head towards the stimuli.
- Appears – birth
- Disappears – 4 months

Palmar/plantar reflex

Stroking the palmar surface of the palm/sole results in the baby grasping the object placed in their hand.
- Appears – birth
- Disappears – 4 months

Stepping

Stimulation of the dorsum of the foot by bringing it into contact with the edge of a table results in the baby stepping onto the table.
- Appears – birth
- Disappears – 6 weeks

Moro

Sudden slight dropping of the babies supported head results in symmetrical extension of the arms and opening of the hands, followed by adduction of the arms.
- Appears – birth
- Disappears – 4 months

Tonic neck reflex

The head is turned to one side when the child is supine. The child develops a 'fencing posture' with extension of the arm that the head is facing and flexion of the contralateral arm and leg.
- Appears – 1 month
- Disappears – 6 months

Downward parachute response

Hold the child in vertical suspension 30 cm above bed and suddenly lower to land on feet. The lower limbs will extent and abduct on landing.
- Appears – 6 months

Forward parachute response

Hold child in prone suspension and suddenly lower head towards bed. The child's upper limbs will abduct to protect themselves.
- Appears – 10 months

4. Fine motor and vision
   - These are examined together
   - Tests include: fixing on face, fixing and following object, grasping, type of hand grip (palmar, scissor, pincer), transferring objects hand-to-hand and hand-to-mouth, picking up small objects, pointing, casting.
5. Hearing and speech
   - This is the most difficult to assess and often you will have to resort to asking the child's mother whether she thinks that the child hears properly and how many words the child can say
   - Tests include: response to rattle, babbling, distraction hearing test (done at 8 months), number of words, comprehension
6. Social
   - Social interaction, peek-a-boo, feeding, toilet training, waves bye-bye, dresses self
7. Growth assessment
   - Measure weight, length and OFC and plot on appropriate growth chart

Eye examination

This is a common short case and should be performed well by all candidates. If told to simply 'examine this child's eyes', we would recommend performing a full examination as below. If told to 'look in this child's eyes', then perform fundoscopy only and then ask if a further examination is required.

1. Introduce yourself to both parents and child
2. During the introduction, you should be making a 'mental survey' of the child, looking for any clues, e.g. ex-premature, tremor, goitre, obvious syndrome
3. Inspection of eyes
   - Orbits
     - shape
     - symmetry
   - Eyelids
     - proptosis (need to look from side or above)
     - ptosis
   - Eyes
     - squint (mention now – cover test later)
     - nystagmus
     - coloboma
     - abnormal size
   - Sclerae
     - colour
     - abnormal vessels

- Iris
  - abnormal colour
  - Brushfield spots
  - Kayser–Fleischer rings
  - aniridia
  - cataract
- Pupils
  - Size
- Conjunctivae
4. Visual acuity
   - Important to know that child can see before progressing
   - Test monocular and binocular vision
   - < 3 years – small objects
   - 3–5 years – Stycar matching letters
   - > 5 years – Snellen charts
5. Pupillary reflexes – light and accommodation reflex

Light reflex
- Shine torch into each eye. Look for direct and consensual reflexes
- Afferent fibres pass in optic nerve → lateral geniculate bodies (some fibres cross chiasma) → bilateral Edinger–Westphal nuclei
- Efferent fibres pass from Edinger–Westphal nuclei → right and left ciliary ganglion via 3rd cranial nerve → pupil
- Therefore bilateral pupil constriction seen

Accommodation reflex
- Ask child to look at your finger held well in front of the child
- Bring your finger in closer until it touches the child's nose
- Observe pupils throughout
- Afferent fibres pass in optic nerve → lateral geniculate bodies (some fibres cross chiasma) → both Edinger–Westphal nuclei and convergence centre
- Efferent fibres pass from convergence centre → Edinger–Westphal nuclei → right and left ciliary ganglion via 3rd cranial nerve → pupil
- Therefore bilateral pupil constriction seen

6. Cover test – squints can be described as
   - Convergent – one eye deviates towards nose (esotropia)
   - Divergent – one eye deviates away from nose (exotropia)
   - Manifest – squint present at all times
   - Latent – squint present when affected eye is covered
   - Alternating – squint alternates between eyes
   - Paralytic/non-paralytic

Observation
- Ask the child to look directly at you. Obvious squint?

Corneal reflection
- Hold a torch 30 cm away from the eyes. The reflection of the light on each cornea should be symmetrical (i.e. the reflection should occur on the same part of the cornea). (Beware epicanthic folds – pseudosquint.)

Cover test

Manifest squint
- Ask the child to look at your nose
- Cover up the straight eye – the squinting will straighten and fix on your nose. Remove the cover and the eyes will return to their original position
- Cover up the squinting eye – there is no change in the position of the straight eye; there is no change in the position of the squinting eye, with or without the cover
- The squint can alternate between eyes

Latent squint
- Ask the child to look at your nose; there is no obvious squint
- Cover one eye – the covered eye deviates (convergent or divegent). There is no change in the position of the non-covered eye. On removing the cover the squinting eye returns to a normal position

7. Eye movements – see cranial nerve examination
8. Visual fields – see cranial nerve examination
9. Fundoscopy – candidates should be able to perform this competently and must be able to recognise the retinal appearances of:
   - Optic atrophy
   - Retinitis pigmentosa
   - Papilloedema
   - Cherry red spot

Head examination

This is a common short case. It is unlikely that you would be asked to perform the entire examination but would be stopped once the relevant clinical signs have been demonstrated.

1. Introduce yourself to both parents and child
2. During the introduction, you should be making a 'mental survey' of the child, looking for any clues.
   - Is the child dysmorphic?
   - Does the child have craniosynostosis?
   - Does the child have micro/macrocephaly?

- Does the child have an obvious squint?
- Does the child have any obvious neurological abnormality?
3. Inspection
    - Assess head size
    - Any scars present? (be sure to look behind ears for shunt)
    - Assess position of eyes
    - Inspect ears
        - shape
        - position
        - pre-auricular skin tags/sinus
4. Palpation

Head circumference
- Offer to measure the child's OFC and plot it on a suitable growth chart

Fontanelle

Shape
- Feel for the anterior and posterior fontanelle
- Anterior
    - diamond-shaped
    - closes by 12–18 months
- Posterior
    - triangular-shaped

Palpation
- Comment on – tense, bulging, pulsating, sunken

Size
- Measure size

Sutures
- Feel the sutures
    - ridging – suggests fusion of sutures
    - wide sutures – hypothyroidism, rickets
5. Assessment of head shape – important to know where the cranial sutures are in order to make sense of head shapes
    - Scaphocephaly
        - premature closure of the sagittal suture
        - ↑ A–P diameter, elongated narrow skull
        - normal face
    - Brachycephaly
        - premature closure of both coronal sutures
        - ↓ A–P diameter, short broad skull
    - Plagiocephaly
        - premature closure of one coronal suture
        - unilateral flattening of skull
    - Trigonocephaly
        - premature closure of metopic suture
        - pointed narrow forehead

6. Auscultation – Important to listen to head for murmur. Listen over fontanelle if present. If fontanelle closed listen over eyes and temporal fossae
7. Eyes – A full examination of the eyes is an important part of the head examination and you should ask to do this

Skin examination

It is important to remember that the skin is a large organ and as much of it as possible should be examined. The hair, nails and mucous membranes are part of the skin and should always be included. The examination is not difficult to do and is purely an exercise in description. The examiners will be impressed if you know a few dermatological terms (Table 2).

Table 2   Dermatological terminology

Macule	Area of discolouration, any size, not raised (flat with skin)
Papule	Small (< 5 mm), raised lesion
Petechiae	Haemorrhage in skin (< 1 mm in diameter), non-blanching
Purpura	Haemorrhage in skin (2–10 mm in diameter), non-blanching
Ecchymoses	Large bruise, non-blanching
Vesicle	Small blister (< 5 mm), elevated, fluid-filled
Bullae	Large blister (> 5 mm), elevated, fluid-filled (serum, seropurulent, blood)
Weal	Elevations in skin, due to acute oedema in dermis, surrounding erythematous macule
Pustule	Elevated, pus-filled
Lichenification	Thickened skin, normal lines in skin more apparent

1. Introduce yourself to parent and child
2. Ask the child to take clothes off down to underwear (if appropriate)
3. Make a visual survey of the whole child noting any rash that is present
4. Description of rash
   - Site
     - area of body – limbs, trunk, scalp, palms, soles of feet
     - pattern – sun-exposed areas, flexures, extensor surfaces
   - Appearance
     - distribution – symmetrical, single, multiple, diffuse, scaling, weeping, irritation
     - colour – red, brown, hyper/hypopigmentation (ask for Wood's lamp if altered pigmentation)
     - shape – round, linear, annular, vesicular, pustular, discoid
   - Palpation
     - blanches? i.e. petechial/purpuric?
     - flush with skin?
     - roughened?

5. Nails – Examine the nails of both hands and feet
   - Pitted nails (psoriasis)
   - Leuchonychia (hypoalbuminaemia)
   - Koilonychia (chronic Fe-deficient anaemia)
   - Absent nails (ectodermal dysplasia)
   - Beau's lines (transverse lines due to temporary arrest in growth secondary to illness)
   - Splinter haemorrhages (endocarditis)
6. Hair
   - Alopecia? totalis/areata
   - Hirsuitism?
   - Abnormal hair – Menke's syndrome, white forelock (Waardenburg syndrome)
   - Hypothyroidism – loss/thinning of outer aspect of eyebrows
7. Mucous membranes
   - Ulceration (herpes simplex, Behçet's, Crohn's)
   - Inflammation (Steven-Johnson syndrome

Assessment of growth and nutrition

This is not a commonly asked short case but it appears to be increasing in popularity. Listed below are some of the measures of growth and nutrition commonly used.

Occipitofrontal circumference (OFC)

This is the maximum occipitofrontal diameter in the horizontal plane. Measure with a *non-stretchable tape* three times and take the *largest value*.

Length

This is usually done in children < 2 years old. Two measurers are needed. One holds the child's head straight, up against the fixed headboard. The other holds the legs out straight, with the feet at right angles to the foot-board. The footboard is brought up to meet the feet and the measurement taken. If longitudinal measures are necessary, they should be done at the same time of day, by the same person, using the same equipment on every occasion.

Height

Usually done in children > 2 years old. The child must be barefoot or in thin socks. Ask the child to stand as tall as possible with feet together and heels on the ground. The heels and the back must be in contact with the vertical measure. The child should be asked to look forward with the lower margin of the eye socket and the external auditory meatus in the same plane (*Frankfurt plane*). Gentle pressure is applied upwards on the mastoid processes. The measuring board is brought down so that it rests lightly on the head and the measurement taken. If longitudinal measures are required the same provisos apply as for length.

Mid arm circumference (MAC)

Measure the circumference at the midpoint of the *non-dominant* upper arm, *hanging freely*, halfway between the acromion and the tip of the olecranon process. Measurements should be done using a *non-stretchable tape*, without indenting the skin and made to the nearest 0.1cm.

As a *very* rough guide, simple standard MAC measurements are given below for different age ranges:

Age	MAC
1–2 years	16.00 cm
2–3 years	16.25 cm
3–4 years	16.50 cm
4–5 years	16.75 cm

Triceps skinfold thickness

Measured again at the midpoint of the upper arm, hanging freely using calipers. An average of three values should be taken. Centile charts exist to produce a percentage of expected for age.

Subscapular and superior iliac crest skinfold thickness measurements are also used.

Weight height indices

Several formulae exist to give an overall measure of nutrition:

- Body mass index $= $ Weight (kg)/height $(m)^2$

- Ponderal index $= $ Weight (kg)/height $(m)^3$

- Weight for height (% expected) $= \dfrac{\text{Child's weight}}{\text{Child's height}} \times \dfrac{\text{50th centile height}}{\text{50th centile weight}} \times 100$

- Z scores $= \dfrac{\text{Child's value} - \text{mean value}}{\text{Standard deviation}}$

Short cases

Achondroplasia

Comment on this child's features

He is *disproportionally short* with a normal-sized trunk but shortening of his proximal limbs (rhizomelia). He has *megalocephaly* with *frontal bossing, depressed nasal saddle* and *midface hypoplasia*. There is bowing of the extremities and short stubby fingers of almost equal length (*trident hand*), but no polydactyly. He has flexion contractures of his elbows and hips. He has marked *lumbar lordosis* with mild thoracolumbar kyphosis and a protuberant abdomen. He walks with a *waddling gait* (secondary to the forward tilt of the pelvis caused by lumbar vertebral wedging). The diagnosis is *achondroplasia*.

Notes

- Autosomal dominant (90% due to new mutation – associated with increased paternal age)
- Incidence = 1 : 30 000 live births
- Chromosome 4 (encodes fibroblast growth factor receptor 3)
- The diagnosis is usually made at birth due to the large head and short limbs that give many rolls of soft tissue and transverse skin creases.
- Hydrocephalus may be present, is usually communicating and secondary to obstruction to the flow of cerebrospinal fluid from narrowing of the foramen magnum
- Lumbar spinal cord compression may occur causing paraplegia in the lower limbs
- Intelligence and fertility are normal
- The umbilicus is the midpoint of the body and the expected average final height is approximately 130 cm. Specific growth charts for achondroplasia should be used

X-ray

- Skull X-ray
  - large vault
  - frontal bossing
  - shortened base
  - shallow sella turcica
- Limb bones
  - long bones short and thick
  - splaying of metaphyseal ends of long bones

- Vertebrae
  - vertebral bodies small and cuboidal with posterior scalloping and some anterior wedging
  - narrow interpeduncular spaces due to thickening of vertebral pedicles resulting in narrowing of the spinal canal
- Pelvis
  - narrow sacrum
  - small square iliac wings (elephant ear)
  - pelvic inlet wide (champagne glass appearance)
  - narrow sciatic notches
  - flat acetabular roofs

Differential diagnosis

Hypochondroplasia
- Autosomal dominant, normal facies
- Short limbs (proximal)

Ellis–van Creveld syndrome
- Autosomal recessive, normal facies
- Hypoplastic nails and teeth
- Atrioseptal heart defect
- Short long bones (distal)
- Polydactyly of fingers and toes

Angelman's syndrome

Comment on this girl's appearance

This young girl has a *jerky ataxia* affecting all 4 limbs. She walks with a *wide-based gait* and she appears to have *microcephaly*, although I would like to confirm this by measuring her head circumference and plotting it on a growth chart. She has frequent excited *clapping of her hands* and *paroxysmal laughter*. I would like to undertake formal assessment of her development, but I do suspect from initial observations that she does have developmental delay. I think she has *Angelman's syndrome*.

Notes

- Male = Female
- EEG – characteristic spike and wave 2 Hz and 5–6 Hz activity uninfluenced by eye opening (most useful investigation)

Genetics

1. 75% – interstitial deletion of the proximal part of the short arm of chromosome 15. The deletion arises from the maternally inherited chromosome 15 (cf. Prader–Willi syndrome see page 171). This is known as *genomic imprinting*, i.e. genetic information expressed differently depending on the parent of origin
2. 2–3% – are found not to have a chromosome deletion but to have inherited two normal chromosome 15s from their father – *paternal uniparental disomy*
3. 5% – chromosome re-arrangments from the mother
4. 15% – no detectable abnormality of genetic material

Features

- Developmental delay
- Fits
- Prominent lower jaw
- Wide mouth
- Frequent tongue thrusting
- Hooked nose
- Blond hair
- Hypotonia
- Absence of choroid pigment and blue eyes

Aortic stenosis

Examine this child's cardiovascular system

This child is pink in air with no evidence of cardiovascular distress and no finger clubbing. Heart rate is 100 per minute, of small volume and slow-rising (*plateau pulse*). The apex beat is not displaced at the 4th intercostal space in the mid-clavicular line and is forceful in character. Palpation over the aortic region (2nd intercostal space, right sternal edge) demonstrates a *systolic thrill* and pulsation is also felt in the *supra-sternal notch*. Auscultation reveals the 1st and 2nd heart sounds, although the 2nd is quiet. There is a harsh *ejection systolic murmur* heard loudest over the aortic region with *radiation up into the neck*. To complete my examination I would look for evidence of cardiac failure (hepatomegaly, peripheral and pulmonary oedema) and measure the blood pressure (decreased pulse pressure). This child has *aortic stenosis*.

Notes

Causes
- Congenital aortic stenosis
- Bicuspid aortic valve
- Hypertrophic obstructive cardiomyopathy
- William's syndrome (see page 230)
- Rheumatic fever (rare)

Auscultation may reveal an ejection click as the aortic valve opens and reversal of the 2nd heart sounds (i.e. the pulmonary valve closes before the aortic valve) if the stenosis is severe. The systolic murmur becomes more prolonged with increased severity.

Investigation

- CXR – smallish heart (because hypertrophy not dilatation) with prominent dilated ascending aorta (post-stenotic dilatation)
- ECG – left ventricular hypertrophy +/– strain, left atrial delay
- Echocardiography
- Angiography – a systolic gradient of over 50–60 mmHg between the left ventricle and aorta at rest with a normal cardiac output requires valvotomy or surgery

Children with aortic stenosis and HOCM should be discouraged from participating in competitive sports.

Ataxia

Assess this boy's cerebellar function

On inspection, this boy has *nystagmus* on lateral gaze. He has a *jerky tremor* of his upper limbs and has difficulty in doing fine co-ordinated hand movements such as building bricks or writing. He cannot perform a finger–nose or heel–shin test (*dysmetria*) and cannot repeatedly pat the back of one hand with the other at speed (*dysdiadokinesia*). When he walks it is with a *broad-based gait* and he has great difficulty walking heel-to-toe. Romberg's sign is negative. His speech is slow and slurred (*scanning dysarthria*). He is generally *hypotonic* and has depressed tendon reflexes but he does demonstrate *pendular knee jerks*. He has *cerebellar ataxia*.

Notes

- Ataxia – abnormalities in executing voluntary movements at the required rate, distance and force

Acute ataxia

Causes

1. Intoxication
   - Most common cause
   - Alcohol, phenytoin, piperazine ('worm wobble'), lead
2. Infection
   - Bacterial – cerebellar abscess, meningitis
   - Viral – encephalitis, meningitis
3. Acute cerebellar ataxia of childhood
   - Seen 1–3 weeks post viral illness (URTI)
   - Affects children aged 1–2 years
   - Aetiology: influenzae A and B, echovirus, coxsackie, mumps, poliomyelitis, herpes simplex, varicella
   - CSF – 10–100 white cells and ↑ protein
   - Recovery within 2 months
4. Structural lesions
   - Cerebellar tumour, head injury
5. ↑ ICP
6. Seizure
7. Hysteria
8. Hypoglycaemia
9. Migraine
10. 'Dancing eye' syndrome (myoclonic encephalopathy of infancy)

Investigation
- Cranial imaging
- Viral titres
- Urine for toxicology screen
- LP

Chronic ataxia

1. Posterior fossa tumour (medulloblastoma, astrocytoma)
2. Cerebral palsy
3. Hydrocephalus
4. Ataxia telangiectasia – see page 42
5. Metabolic
   - Leucodystrophies (metachromatic, Krabbe)
   - Batten's disease
   - Refsum's syndrome
   - Abetalipoproteinaemia
   - Tay–Sach's disease – see page 53
   - Wilson's disease – see page 216
6. Friedrich's ataxia

Ataxia telangiectasia (Louis-Bar syndrome)

> **Comment on this boy's appearance and examine his cerebellar function**
>
> This young boy has numerous *telangiectasia* on his conjunctivae and face in a butterfly distribution. He walks with a *wide-based gait*. He is unable to do the *finger–nose test* and has impairment of rapidly alternating hand movements (*dysdiadochokinesis*). His hand movements are clumsy and jerky (*dyssynergia*). He has *cerebellar ataxia*. From his facial appearance and ataxia this boy's diagnosis is *ataxia telangiectasia*.

Notes

- Autosomal recessive
- Chromosome 11
- Multisystemic disorder
- Early development normal
- Cerebellar ataxia begins age 1–2 years
- Progressive neurological deterioration – most are wheelchair-bound by 10 years of age
- Telangiectasia develop on bulbar conjunctivae and other areas exposed to sunlight (ear pinnae, nares, flexures of elbows/knees) after age 3–5 years.

Immunity

- Defect in cellular and humoral immunity seen
- Recurrent upper respiratory tract infections – nasal sinus, middle ear, lungs → bronchiectasis
- ↓ IgA, ↓ IgE, ↓ IgM, ↓ IgG_2, ↓ IgG_4
- CXR – absent thymic shadow
- Tonsils – hypoplastic

Malignancy

- Develop in 33%
- Lymphoma, sarcoma, lymphosarcoma, leukaemia, cerebellar neoplasms, ovarian dysgerminoma, gastric carcinoma
- Defect in DNA repair mechanism – high incidence of chromosomal breaks
- ↑ serum α-fetoprotein

Other

- Growth retardation
- Developmental delay
- Gonadal atrophy in both sexes
- Glucose intolerance

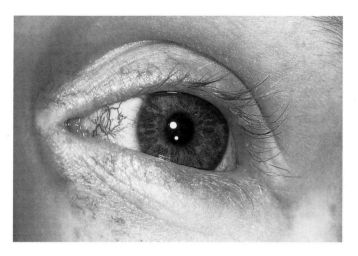

Fig. 1 Classical appearance of the cornea in ataxia telangectasia

Atrial septal defect

Examine this boy's cardiovascular system

This young boy is pink and has no cardiorespiratory distress. On inspection of his hands there is no evidence of clubbing or peripheral cyanosis. His pulse is 85 beats per minute and is of normal rhythm, character and volume. He has no brachial–brachial or brachio–femoral delay and his blood pressure in his right arm is 80/50. His apex pulse is in the 5th left intercostal space and there are no thrills or heaves. Auscultation of his chest reveals an *ejection systolic murmur* in the pulmonary area with *fixed splitting of the second heart sound*. I would conclude my examination by listening to his lung bases and palpating his abdomen for evidence of hepatosplenomegaly. The diagnosis is *atrial septal defect*.

Notes – Ostium secundum ASD

- Accounts for 8% of congenital heart defects
- 3 females : 1 male
- Occurs due to failure of closure of the foramen ovale
- Associated syndromes – Holt–Oram syndrome (see page 120)

Clinical
- Children are usually asymptomatic
- Adults develop pulmonary hypertension, heart failure, atrial arrhythmias

Pulse
- Normal, no thrill

Heart sounds
- S1 – normal
- S2 – wide fixed splitting (due to conduction delay and delayed closure of the pulmonary valve)

Murmur
- Ejection systolic murmur in 2nd left intercostal space (due to increased blood through a normal pulmonary valve)
- Mid-diastolic murmur in 4th right intercostal space (due to increased blood through normal tricuspid valve) if pulmonary blood flow is $2 \times$ systemic blood flow

Chest X-ray
- Normal or cardiomegaly with prominent right atrium and pulmonary artery

ECG

- Sinus rhythm
- Right axis deviation
- Incomplete RBBB
- RsR' in V1 and V4R

Treatment

- Surgical repair

Basic life support

This is becoming a frequent short case and it is not uncommon for a candidate to be asked to resuscitate a baby mannequin. Basic life support is outlined as in the most recent edition of the *Advanced Paediatric Life Support* book. It is imperative that the candidate be able to recite the cardiac algorithms and be able to talk through the management of all emergencies.

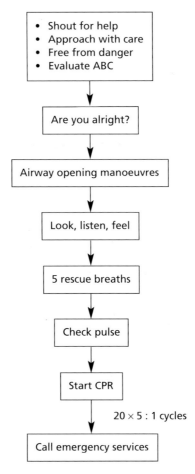

Look at this boy's face and tell me what you think:

This boy demonstrates facial asymmetry at rest with *loss of the naso-labial fold* and an *inability to close his eye* or *wrinkle his forehead* on the left side. He has drooping of the corner of his mouth and his speech is slurred. Attempting to smile demonstrates an inability to lift the left side of his mouth. He has tears running down his face from the left eye. There is no evidence of *herpes zoster* infection of the left ear (Ramsay Hunt syndrome) and systemic blood pressure is normal. He is likely to have a *Bell's palsy*, but I would like to exclude other pathologies by radiological imaging of the middle ear (e.g. nasopharyngeal rhabdomyosarcoma).

Notes

- Idiopathic lower motor neurone facial nerve paralysis
- Frequently preceded by an upper respiratory tract illness
- Onset of weakness often heralded by pain around the sternomastoid
- Associated with more serious illnesses including mumps, otitis media, herpes zoster and Lyme disease (*Borrelia burgdorferi*)
- Involvement of the branches of the facial nerve can cause other symptoms
  - impaired lacrimation – greater superficial petrosal nerve
  - loss of taste of the anterior two-thirds of the tongue (50%) – chorda tympani
  - hyperacussis – nerve to the stapedius muscle

Treatment

- Corticosteroids or ACTH given within 3 days of onset (presumably to reduce oedema within the facial canal) are advocated by some neurologists, but not all!
- Eye care to prevent corneal damage

Prognosis

- If complete recovery is likely, some return of facial movement should occur within the first 4 weeks
- Better prognosis in children
- Faulty re-innervation can occur resulting in 'crocodile tears' (crying on eating) or eye closure on pursing the lips

Differential diagnosis

- Hypertension – due to haemorrhage or oedema within the facial canal
- Birth trauma – with or without forceps delivery
- Local tumours – sarcomas or metastases of the middle ear
- Melkersson's syndrome – recurrent unilateral or bilateral facial nerve palsy associated with facial oedema, most commonly the upper lip

N.B. Bilateral facial nerve palsy seen in Guillain–Barré syndrome, Moebius syndrome, polio, diphtheria, sarcoid and Lyme disease.

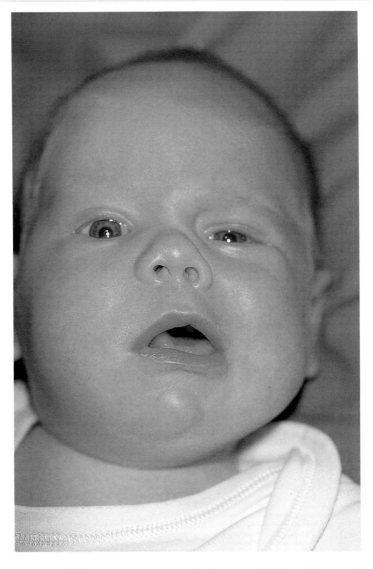

Fig. 2 Right-sided lower motor neurone facial nerve palsy in an infant aged 3 months

Bronchopulmonary dysplasia

What do you think about this 3-month-old infant?

The most obvious findings on initial examination are that this infant is *oxygen-dependent*, he does not have much subcutaneous fat, he appears small for his age and he has *scaphocephaly*. Respiratory system examination demonstrates a saturation of 92% with 0.5 l/min oxygen being administered via nasal cannulae. There are several scars on the anterior and lateral chest wall (previous chest drain insertion for pneumothorax). Respiratory rate is 60 breaths per minute with subcostal and intercostal *recession*. Auscultation reveals fine *inspiratory crepitations* throughout the lung fields and an occasional expiratory wheeze. He has a 2 finger-breadth smoothly enlarged liver below the right subcostal margin (secondary to hyperinflation and/or a degree of right-sided heart failure). I would like to plot his weight, length and head circumference on the appropriate centile chart. This boy is an ex-premature baby with *bronchopulmonary dysplasia*. I would like to conclude my examination by looking for other potential stigmata of prematurity including patent ductus arteriosus (PDA), retinopathy of prematurity and finally undertake a full developmental assessment.

Notes

- X-rays
  - areas of hyperlucency from cystic changes and hyperinflation
  - streaky infiltration secondary to interstitial oedema, mucosal hyperplasia, fibrosis and alveolar collapse
  - cardiomegaly and increased vascular lung markings from pulmonary hypertension or coexistent PDA

Differential diagnosis

- Wilson–Mikity syndrome – absence of features of hyaline membrane disease in the immediate newborn period with development of respiratory distress towards the end of the first week of life

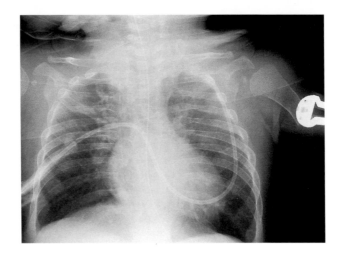

Fig. 3 X-ray appearances in BPD

Cataract

Look in this girl's eyes

On examination of this young girl's eyes she demonstrates bilateral densities of the lenses. There is bilateral *absence of the red reflex* on fundoscopy and I am unable to visualise the retinae. She has *roving nystagmus*, she does not fix on my face or other objects and I suspect that she is *blind*. She does not have stigmata of congenital infection (congenital varicella – limb hypoplasia/scarring, cortical atrophy; congenital toxoplasmosis – hydrocephaly, microphthalmia, hepatosplenomegaly; congenital rubella – growth retardation, microcephaly, deafness). I would like to measure her head circumference and undertake a more extensive examination to see if I can discover the cause of her *cataracts* (see below).

Notes

- Cataract – opacity of the crystalline lens
- Can be unilateral/bilateral, partial/complete
- Variation in extent, position, shape and density

Aetiology

1. Idiopathic
2. Congenital – autosomal dominant, autosomal recessive, X-linked
3. Intrauterine infection – rubella, varicella, toxoplasmosis, syphilis
4. Trauma
5. Drug-induced – long-term corticosteroids
6. Metabolic
   - Galactosaemia, hypocalcaemia, hypoglycaemia, diabetes mellitus
   - Lowe's oculo-cerebro-renal dystrophy
7. Syndromes
   - Down's syndrome – see page 88
   - Turner's syndrome – see page 221
   - Crouzon's syndrome – see page 73
   - Apert's syndrome – see page 73
   - Rubenstein–Taybi syndrome – see page 187
   - Ellis–van Creveld syndrome – see page 37
   - Hurler's syndrome – see page 123
8. Others
   - Post-radiation
   - Myotonic dystrophy – see page 152

- Atopic dermatitis
- Congenital ichthyosis
- Wilson's disease
- 2° to lens dislocation
  - Marfan's syndrome – see page 147
  - Homocystinuria

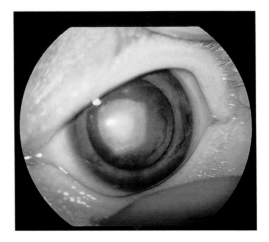

Fig. 4 Cataract

Cherry red spot

Examine this boy's retina

Examination of this young boy's retina reveals a small red spot at the macula (lateral to the optic disc) surrounded by a pale halo in both eyes. The rest of the retina appears normal. This child has *cherry red spots*.

Notes

Cherry red spots are seen when there is accumulation of abnormal substances in the retinal ganglion cells. Because the fovea is not covered with ganglion cells it appears red. Distended retinal ganglion cells appear pale.

Cherry red spots are seen in:

1. Tay–Sachs disease
2. Niemann–Pick disease
3. Farber's disease
4. Sandhoff's disease
5. Sialidosis I and II

Tay–Sachs disease (G_{M2} gangliosidosis Type 1)

- Autosomal recessive
- Chromosome 15
- Gene frequency 1:25 in Ashkenazi Jews
- Deficiency of β-hexoaminidase A
- Accumulation of G_{M2} ganglioside in lysosomes of CNS only and therefore the disease is confined to the CNS
- Presents by age 6 months with decreased eye contact, hyperacusis (marked startle response to noise), retinal cherry red spots and macrocephaly
- By 12 months of age children are blind, hypotonic and have developmental delay
- Death by 2–4 years of age from respiratory failure
- No treatment available

Niemann–Pick disease (Types A, B, C, D)

- Autosomal recessive
- Type A most common and severe

- Deficiency of sphingomyelinase resulting in accumulation of sphingomyelin in lysosomes of the reticular-endothelial system and CNS
- Presents age 3 months with failure to thrive, hepatosplenomegaly, developmental delay and retinal cherry red spots
- Death age 1–4 years (respiratory failure)

Farber's disease

- Autosomal recessive
- Deficiency of ceramidase resulting in accumulation of ceramide in tissues
- Onset in the first few months of life
- Presents with painful joints, subcutaneous nodules and retinal cherry red spots.
- Death in first year of life from respiratory failure

Sandhoff's disease (G_{M2} gangliosidosis Type 2)

- Autosomal recessive
- Deficiency of β-hexoaminidase A and B
- Onset aged 6–9 months
- Clinical picture similar to Tay–Sachs disease
- Hepatosplenomegaly seen

Sialidosis I and II

- Autosomal recessive
- Deficiency of N-acetylneuraminidase (sialidase)

Child with a limp

This child has a limp. Please assess

On inspection this tall, *overweight teenage* boy appears well and is *afebrile*. On examination of his gait he appears to have a limp affecting his right hip. I would like to ask him if his hip is painful before proceeding. On inspection of his right hip there is no evidence of swelling or erythema. The joint is not warm to the touch. He has *limitation of abduction, external rotation and internal rotation* of the right hip on both passive and active movement. I would like to make a full examination of his knee, ankle, feet and shoes. My working diagnosis in a child of this age is *slipped upper femoral epiphysis*.

Notes

Causes of limp in children:

1. Irritable hip (transient synovitis)
   - Commonest cause of acute onset hip pain and limp in children
   - Age of onset 2–10; male > female
   - Aetiology – unknown but 70% have viral URTI 7–14 days prior to limp
   - FBC, ESR – normal X-ray may show widening of joint space
   - Resolves in 7–10 days
2. Trauma
3. Developmental dysplasia of hip (DDH)/congenital dislocation of hip (CDH)
   - Ranges from dislocatable hip to a dislocated hip. Early diagnosis and treatment is essential
   - Incidence = 2 : 1000; unilateral > bilateral
   - Associations
     - increased family history
     - breech presentation
     - oligohydramnios
     - spina bifida
   - Clinical
     - asymmetrical skin creases
     - shortening of limb
   - Investigation
     - examination – Ortolani/Barlow's test
     - ultrasound – newborn to 3 months old
     - X-ray – Child > 3 months

- Treatment
  - orthopaedic management
  - positioning of hips (e.g. Pavlik harness, hip spica)
4. Septic arthritis/osteoarthritis – see page 201
5. Juvenile chronic arthritis – see page 134
6. Slipped upper femoral epiphysis (adolescent coxa vara)
   - Peak age of incidence 10–15; M > F; 20% bilateral
   - Thought to be due to an imbalance of growth hormone : sex hormone
   - Associated with obesity, tall stature, gonadal immaturity
   - Presents with painful hip, thigh, knee
   - No swelling
   - Limitation of abduction, extension and internal rotation
   - May cause compromise of blood flow to femoral head
   - X-ray – slipped capital epiphysis downwards and backwards
7. Perthe's disease
   - Idiopathic avascular necrosis of femoral head
   - Peak age of incidence 5–10; 5 males : 1 female; 20% bilateral
   - Aetiology – unknown. Familial tendency
   - Presents with painful/painless limp and decreased range of movement
   - Leads to irregularity and fragmentation of the femoral head
   - FBC, ESR – normal
8. Henoch–Schönlein purpura – see page 112
9. Haemarthrosis – haemophilia A and B

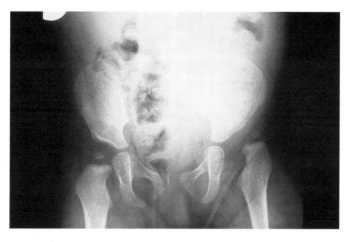

Fig. 5 X ray showing developmental dysplasia of left hip

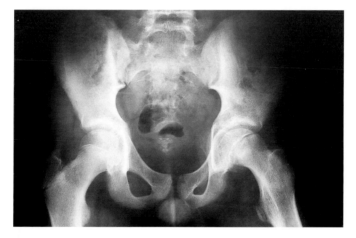

Fig. 6 Left-sided slipped upper femoral epiphysis

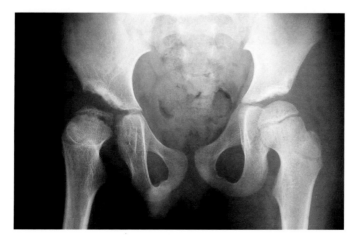

Fig. 7 Perthe's disease of the right hip

Clubbing

Examine this girl's hands

On examination of this girl's hands she has loss of the angle between the nailbed and the finger. There is increased rounding of the fingers in both directions and increased softening of the nailbed. I would like to examine her toenails. This young girl has finger *clubbing*. To investigate the cause I would like to make a full examination of her cardiovascular, respiratory and abdominal systems.

Notes

Clubbing doesn't appear until > 1 year of age (except with congenital clubbing!). Appears in the thumbs first.

Causes

1. Cardiovascular
   - Congenital cyanotic heart disease
   - Subacute infective endocarditis
2. Respiratory
   - Bronchiectasis
   - Lung abscess
   - Empyema
   - Pulmonary TB
   - Cystic fibrosis
   - Pulmonary fibrosis
   - Pulmonary haemosiderosis
   - Pleural and mediastinal tumours
3. Gastrointestinal
   - Ulcerative colitis
   - Crohn's disease
   - Biliary cirrhosis
   - Chronic active hepatitis
4. Miscellaneous
   - Congenital
   - Atrial myxoma
   - Leiomyoma
   - Thalassaemia
   - Hodgkin's disease
   - HIV infection

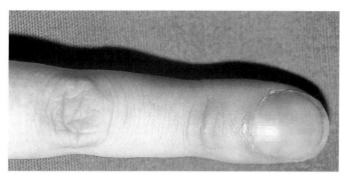

Fig. 8 Clubbing

Coarctation of the aorta

Examine this girl's cardiovascular system

This small, 13–year-old girl is not centrally cyanosed and has no cardio-respiratory distress. She has no finger clubbing, splinter haemorrhages or peripheral cyanosis. Her pulse is 75 beats per minute and is of normal rhythm, character and volume. She has *radio-femoral delay* and the *femoral pulses are of reduced volume*. Her brachial pulses are normal. Her blood pressure is *160/110*. Inspecting her chest, I note that she has *widely spaced nipples* and a *webbed neck*. She has a *left lateral thoracotomy scar*. The cardiac impulse is heaving and the apex is in the 5th left intercostal space. There is a *systolic thrill* present over the scapula. She has a *systolic murmur* heard loudest over the left sternal border that radiates through to the back, loudest between the scapula. Her lung fields are clear and she has no peripheral oedema. I would like to palpate her abdomen for evidence of hepato-splenomegaly.

The diagnosis is *coarctation of the aorta* in a girl with *Turner's syndrome*. The left lateral thoracotomy scar probably represents a previous coarctation repair.

Notes

- Coarctation accounts for 6% of congenital heart disease
- 3 males : 1 female
- 15% of girls with Turner's syndrome have a coarctation (50% have other cardiac anomalies including VSD, mitral valve abnormalities, aortic stenosis)
- Hypertension result from decreased renal perfusion and increased renin secretion
- CXR
  - penetrated X-ray – Figure 3 shape to aorta (1st bulge – aorta above coarctation, 2nd – post-stenotic dilatation)
  - children > 6 years old demonstrate rib notching due to collateral vessels
  - ECG – Left ventricular hypertrophy

Treatment

- Surgical repair (end-to-end, subclavian flap, graft)
- Mortality < 1%
- Complications – re-coarctation, spinal cord infarction

Coarctation in the newborn child

- Presents in first few days when the ductus closes
- Presentation – dyspnoea, collapse, poor peripheral perfusion, acute renal failure, hepatomegaly
- CXR – cardiomegaly, plethoric lung fields
- ECG – right ventricular hypertrophy

Treatment

- Acute resuscitation – prostaglandin infusion, correction of acidosis, hypocalcaemia, hypoglycaemia; dopamine infusion
- Surgical repair

N.B. Right lateral thoracotomy scar = shunt procedure, TOF repair
Left lateral thoracotomy scar = shunt procedure, pulmonary banding, coarctation repair, PDA repair

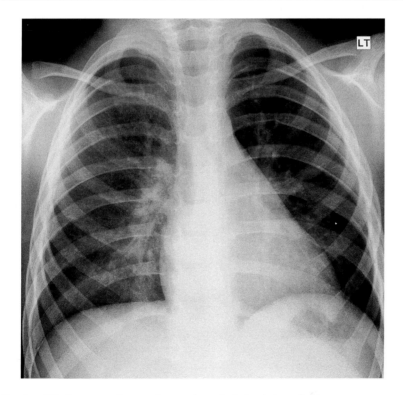

Fig. 9   CXR demonstrating cardiomegaly and plethoric lung fields

Coeliac disease (gluten enteropathy)

> ## Examine this boy's abdomen
>
> This rather *miserable* boy is *pale*. He appears *short* but I would like to confirm this by plotting his height (and weight) on a growth chart. He has a *protuberant abdomen* and *wasted buttocks* and *legs*. Examination of his abdomen is otherwise unremarkable. The diagnosis is *coeliac disease*.

Notes

- Results from sensitivity of the proximal small bowel to α-gliadin, the alcohol-soluble fraction of gluten
- Gluten present in wheat, rye, barley and oats (not maize and corn)
- Presents most commonly aged 6–12 months (time when gluten introduced to diet) but can present at any age after weaning, throughout life

Epidemiology

- Incidence = 1 : 2000 in UK/USA, 1 in 200 in Galway, Ireland
- 2 females : 1 male; 10% of cases are familial
- Rare in Blacks and Asians
- HLA-DR4 in 100%, HLA-DQW2 in 98%, HLA-DR3 in > 90%, HLA-DR7 in > 90%, HLA B8 +ve in 85%

Aetiology is unknown but it is thought to have an immunological basis (cellular- and humoral-mediated).

Other features

- Diarrhoea (bulky, pale, greasy, offensive, and difficult to flush)
- Failure to thrive
- Hypotonia
- Delayed puberty
- 2° lactose intolerance due to damaged brush border
- Rickets (vitamin D deficiency secondary to fat malabsorption – look for rickety rosary and splaying at the wrist)

Investigations

- Anaemia (Fe deficiency, folate deficiency occasionally)

- Decreased fat-soluble vitamins (vitamins A, D, E, K)
- ↑ Prothrombin time (due to vitamin K malabsorption – check before biopsy)
- Hypoalbuminaemia – loss of protein through the gut wall and decreased hepatic synthesis from malnutrition)
- ↑ Faecal fat (normal child excretes 5–10% of ingested fat, coeliac child excretes > 15%) – do fat microscopy

Serology

- IgG anti-gliadin antibodies (sensitivity 90–100%, specificity 60–95%)
- IgA anti-gliadin antibodies (sensitivity 60–100%, specificity 86–100%)
- IgG anti-gliadin antibodies present in 10% of normal children
- IgG & IgA anti-reticulin antibodies (sensitivity 50–60%)
- IgG & IgA anti-endomysium antibodies (sensitivity 50–100%)

Antibodies

- Preliminary screening, monitoring treatment and detecting non-compliance to treatment

Diagnosis

- Classical biopsy findings
- Full clinical remission after withdrawal of gluten from diet

The 3 biopsy sequence (1st = diagnosis, 2nd = after gluten exclusion, 3rd = relapse after challenge) is not necessary if first biopsy shows classical changes, clinical improvement occurs with gluten-free diet and antibodies elevated at diagnosis return to normal after gluten exclusion.

Histology

- Short/absent villi
- Crypt hyperplasia
- Abnormal cuboidal enterocytes
- Lymphoid cell infiltration
- Intra-epithelial lymphocytes
- Plasma cells in lamina propria

Differential diagnosis of subtotal/total villous atrophy

- Gastroenteritis (postenteritis syndrome)
- Cow's milk protein intolerance
- Giardiasis

Associations

- Dermatitis herpetiformis
- Diabetes mellitus (IDDM)
- Thyroid disease
- Arthritis
- Down's syndrome (increased incidence of autoimmune disorders)

Treatment

- Gluten-free diet for life
- Severely ill patients with coeliac crisis can be treated with corticosteroids
- Relaxation of diet in adults causes malaise, anaemia, infertility and osteomalacia
- Failure to comply with diet increases the risk of small bowel malignant T-cell lymphoma and carcinoma of the jejunum, oesophagus and rectum

Coloboma

Examine this boy's eyes

On inspection this child has a *wedge-shaped absence of the iris* of both eyes. The pupils appear normal. Pupillary reflexes, visual fields and eye movements are normal. I would like to assess his vision using a Snellen chart. To conclude my examination I would like to perform fundoscopy. The diagnosis is bilateral *coloboma of the iris*.

Notes

Coloboma can involve the iris, lens, retina or eyelid. They may occur in isolation or as part of a syndrome.

Syndromes involving coloboma

1. CHARGE association
(N.B. 'association' – combination of abnormalities which occur together more often than expected by chance.)

   Coloboma – iris or retina
   Heart defect – tetralogy of Fallot, endocardial cushion defect, VSD, ASD
   Atresia choanal
   Retarded growth
   Genital abnormality
   Ear abnormality – protruding ears, overfolded helices/deafness

   Also seen – developmental delay, renal anomalies, tracheoesophageal fistula, micrognathia, cleft lip and palate, hypogonadism, exomphalos.

2. Goldenhar association (oculoauriculovertebral dysplasia)
   • Aetiology – failure of migration of neural crest cells into the 1st and 2nd branchial arches in the 4th week of fetal life
   • Features
     • facial – frontal bossing, facial asymmetry, mandibular hypoplasia, maxillary hypoplasia
     • ears – preauricular skin tags, microtia, absent external auditory canals, conductive hearing loss
     • eye – epibulbar dermoids, unilateral *coloboma*, microphthalmia
     • vertebral – spina bifida, hemivertebrae, synostoses, cuneiform vertebrae
     • cardiac – Fallot's, VSD

3. 'Cat eye' syndrome
   - Defect – chromosome 22
   - Features
     - renal agenesis
     - down-slanting palpebral fissures
     - cardiac defects
     - anal atresia
     - inferior *coloboma* of iris
     - developmental delay
4. Wolf–Hirschhorn syndrome
   - Defect – chromosomal deletion (4p-)
   - Features
     - *colobomata*
     - hypertelorism
     - low set ears
     - flat nasal bridge
     - cardiac and renal anomalies
     - developmental delay
     - facial features resemble Greek helmet
     - death in early childhood
5. Patau syndrome (trisomy 13)
   - Incidence = 1 : 6000. Most cases due to non-disjunction
   - Features
     - severe developmental delay
     - failure to thrive
     - seizures
     - microcephaly
     - cleft lip and palate
     - midline scalp defects
     - microphthalmia
     - holoprosencephaly
     - *colobomata*
     - congenital heart defects (VSD)
     - polycystic kidney
     - post-axial polydactyly
     - exomphalos
     - 90% dead by 1 year of age

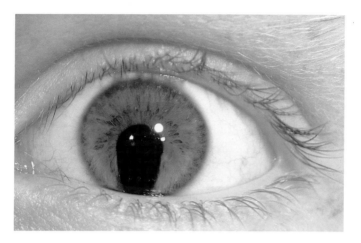

Fig. 10 Coloboma

Constipation

> ## Comment on this 14-year-old girl's appearance and examine her abdomen
>
> This girl has dry, sparse hair and is missing the outer part of her eyebrows. Her skin is dry and she appears overweight, although I would like to confirm this using an appropriate growth chart. On inspection of her abdomen it appears mildly distended and on palpation I can feel a hard irregular mass in her left iliac fossa. I think this girl has co-existent *hypothyroidism* and *constipation*. I would like to look for other evidence of autoimmune disease (vitiligo, urine dipstick for glucose), record her heart rate (bradycardia) and check her thyroid function tests (and perform an abdominal X-ray – contentious!) to confirm the diagnoses.

Notes

Constipation is the passage of infrequent and sometimes painful stools and is a symptom rather than a disease. Remember – one man's constipation is another man's diarrhoea!

Aetiology

Non-organic
- Functional – 95% of cases

Organic
- Nutritional
  - low dietary fibre
  - poor fluid intake
  - excess cow's milk
- Anatomical
  - Hirschsprung's disease
  - anal stenosis/stricture
  - rectal fissure/abscess
- Drugs
  - lead poisoning
  - opiates
  - antacids (containing calcium or aluminium)
- Metabolic
  - hypercalcaemia
  - hypokalaemia
  - renal tubular acidosis

- diabetes insipidus
- rickets
- cystic fibrosis (meconium ileus equivalent)
- Neuromuscular
  - infantile botulism
  - myotonic dystrophy
  - spinal cord lesions

Hirschsprung's disease

- Incidence = 1:5000
- Aetiology – absence of ganglion cells in the myenteric plexuses (Meissner and Auerbach) due to failure of migration from the neural crest
- History – delayed passage of meconium, constipation from birth, marked abdominal distention

Short-segment Hirschsprung's
- 5 males : 1 female
- Affects rectum and rectosigmoid

Long-segment Hirschsprung's
- 1 male : 1 female
- Extends above sigmoid
- 10–15% of cases have Down's syndrome
- In long-standing cases the mucosa of the affected area becomes thin and inflamed (enterocolitis) → perforation in some cases

Investigation
- Abdominal X-ray → distension
- Rectal suction biopsy (1 and 3 cm above dentate line) → absence of ganglion cells in submucosal plexus, excessive acetylcholinesterase in abnormal nerves

Treatment
- Colostomy
- Anorectal pull through

Cornelia de Lange syndrome

What do you think Rachel has (spot diagnosis)?

Her facial features are suggestive of *Cornelia de Lange syndrome*. She has *synophyrs* (eyebrows meeting in the midline), *microcephaly*, a long philtrum and a short nose with *anteverted nostrils*. Looking more widely, I note that she has generalised *hirsuitism* and has several anatomical abnormalities of her upper limbs (absent ulna, single palmar crease, absent fingers, proximally placed thumbs). She has *developmental delay*. All these features are consistent with the diagnosis.

Notes

- Inheritance – uncertain. Milder cases have been reported as autosomal dominant
- Other
  - long, curved eyelashes
  - microphthalmia
  - low set ears
  - micrognathia
  - feeding difficulties
  - cutis marmorata
  - congenital diaphragmatic, inguinal, hiatus and umbilical herniae
  - cryptorchidism in boys
  - gastrointestinal abnormalities
  - thrombocytopenia

Features

- Characteristically low birth weight
- Short stature
- Microcephaly
- Generalised hirsutism

Synonymous names include de Lange syndrome, Brachmann de Lange syndrome and Amsterdam dwarf.

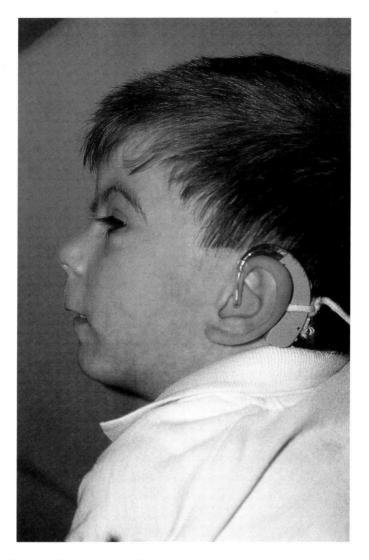

Fig. 11 Cornelia de Lange syndrome

Cradle cap

Examine the scalp of this young baby

On inspection this infant has an erythematous dermatitis with *yellow, greasy, crusty scales* affecting his scalp and eyebrows. His nappy area and flexures are clear. His teeth, nails and hair are normal.

The most common cause of this is seborrhoeic dermatitis ('*cradle cap*') although it is important to exclude other rarer causes such as psoriasis, fungal infection, AIDS and Langerhan's cell histiocytosis (histiocytosis X).

Notes

- Seborrhoeic dermatitis is of unknown cause
- Treatment involves softening of the scales with olive oil and subsequent combing of the hair. Occasionally, topical steroids may be used if there are inflamed areas
- A poor response to treatment should question the diagnosis

Langerhan's cell histiocytosis

Abnormal proliferation of phagocytic histiocytes; three diseases seen:

1. Solitary bone lesion (eosinophilic granuloma)
   - Single lytic bone lesion on X-ray
   - Diagnostic curettage may be curative
   - Other treatments – intracavity steroid injection
2. Multiple bone lesions
   These can occur anywhere. The following triad can occur:
   - multiple lytic skull lesions and soft tissue lesions
   - proptosis
   - diabetes insipidus – granuloma around the pituitary stalk
3. Systemic Langerhan's cell histiocytosis
   - Multisystem disease – involves liver, spleen, lungs, gut, bone marrow, brown papular rash of neck and trunk, seborrhoeic dermatitis of scalp
   - Treatment – chemotherapy

Craniosynostosis

Examine this girl's head

This young girl has an abnormally shaped head that is tall (*turri-cephaly*) with a short A–P diameter (acrocephaly). I would like to measure her occipital-frontal circumference and plot it on a growth chart. I note that she also has *hypoplasia of her midface, shallow orbits, a small nose, hypertelorism, proptosis, strabismus, a prominent jaw, a high arched palate, a flattened occiput* and *syndactyly* of her fingers and toes. The diagnosis is *Apert's syndrome.*

Notes

- Infants are often seen with plagiocephaly that is a result of moulding. It requires only reassurance
- *Craniosynostosis* results from premature closure of one or more of the cranial sutures
- Premature closure of the sagittal suture results in scaphocephaly (elongation of the head in the antero-posterior direction)
- Premature closure of the coronal sutures results in brachycephaly (increase in cranial diameter from left to right, flattened back of head)
- Cranial imaging with X-ray ± CT/MRI are the investigations of choice
- Treatment – reconstructive surgery

Craniosynostosis is seen in isolation and in association with syndromes:

1. Apert's syndrome (acroscaphocephaly)
   - Autosomal dominant
   - Features
     - as above
     - broad thumbs
   - Associated with
     - anal atresia
     - pyloric stenosis
     - congenital heart disease
     - skeletal defects
2. Crouzon's syndrome (craniofacial dysostosis)
   - Autosomal dominant
   - Features
     - premature fusion of coronal, sagittal and lambdoidal sutures
     - frontal bossing
     - shallow orbits

- hypertelorism
- exophthalmos
- hypoplastic maxilla
- beaked parrot-like nose
- low set ears
- conductive hearing loss
- nystagmus
- strabismus
- optic atrophy
- fits
- developmental delay

3. Pfeiffer's syndrome
   - Autosomal dominant
   - Features
     - premature closure of coronal, ± sagittal sutures
     - brachycephaly
     - antimongoloid upslanting palpebral fissures
     - small nose and low nasal bridge
     - broad distal phalanges of thumb and big toe
     - partial syndactyly of 2nd and 3rd fingers
     - normal intelligence

4. Carpenter syndrome
   - Autosomal recessive
   - Features
     - premature closure of coronal, sagittal and lamboid sutures
     - brachycephaly
     - shallow orbital ridges
     - obese
     - lateral displacement of inner canthi
     - hands – brachydactyly with clindodactyly; partial syndactyly

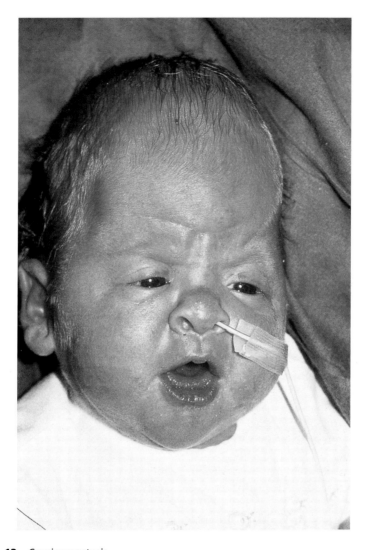

Fig. 12 Craniosynostosis

Crohn's disease

Carry out an abdominal system examination for me

This pale, asthenic 13-year-old boy has *finger clubbing, swollen lips* and *ulceration* of his buccal cavity. Abdominal system examination reveals only several *healed surgical scars*. I would like to look for the presence of *peri-anal skin tags, fissures, fistulae* and *abscesses* which would be further evidence pointing towards the likely diagnosis of *Crohn's disease*. I would also look for extra-intestinal manifestations of inflammatory bowel disease including *erythema nodosum, pyoderma gangrenosum, eye disease* and *arthritis*. Plotting his height and weight on the appropriate centile chart would complete my initial examination.

Notes

- Incidence = 3–7 : 100 000, prevalence = 40 : 100 000
- 1 male : 1 female
- Less common than ulcerative colitis (incidence 6–15 per 100 000)
- 40% present before age 20 years, 20% before 15 years
- Majority present with abdominal pain, altered stool habit and weight loss. Bleeding PR in ~50% (100% in UC)
- Extra-intestinal manifestations common
  - growth failure (85%)
  - arthralgia and arthritis (40%) including ankylosing spondylitis
  - skin (up to 30%) – erythema nodosum and pyoderma gangrenosum
  - finger clubbing (25–60%)
  - urolithiasis (15%)
  - eye (4%) – conjunctivitis, iritis and episcleritis
  - vascular (3%) – arteritis and thromboembolic disease
  - hepatobiliary disease (3%) – fatty change, pericholangitis, cirrhosis
  - miscellaneous (rare) – pericarditis, amyloidosis

Differential diagnosis

- Ulcerative colitis
  - continuous proximally from the rectum and symmetrical involvement around the colonic circumference
  - no skip lesions
  - strictures and fistulae are more common in Crohn's disease

- Ileocaecal tuberculosis
- Behçet's disease
- Amoebic colitis
- NSAID abuse
- Coeliac disease

Cushingoid facies

What can you tell me about this boy's facial appearance?

This 11-year-old boy has a *round face* (is it acceptable to say 'moon' face or fat face in front of the child and family?), *flushed cheeks* and has *acne*. I note that he has a peak flow meter and a salbutamol metered dose inhaler and spacer on his bedside locker. On more general inspection he has *truncal obesity, fine lanugo hair* and *striae* on his anterior abdominal wall and thighs. His limbs are thin and he finds it difficult to stand from squatting down (*proximal myopathy* from chronic corticosteroid use). I would like to go on to examine his respiratory tract system because I think he may be *Cushingoid* as a result of chronic corticosteroid treatment for severe asthma.

I would also like to check his blood pressure (for *hypertension*) dipstick the urine (for glucose, protein), plot his height and weight on a centile chart and look at his eyes (for cataract).

Notes

- Cushing's syndrome is due to increased adrenocortical function
- Cushing's disease is specifically adrenocorticoid excess due to increased pituitary ACTH production (pituitary or hypothalamic lesions)
- Cushingoid is simply a descriptive term for the physical characteristics caused by adrenocorticoid excess from whatever cause
- Features of adrenocorticoid excess
  - 'buffalo hump'
  - thin skin
  - easy bruising (due to capillary fragility)
  - short stature
  - centripetal obesity ('lemon on a cocktail stick')
  - loss of the supraclavicular fossa (normally preserved in other forms of obesity)

N.B. If adrenocortical tumours have significant androgenic secretion, precocious puberty and short-term growth acceleration can be seen. Other androgenic effects include a deepening of the voice, hypertrichosis and acne.

Cushingoid features due to exogenous corticosteroids

- Severe asthma
- Transplantation and immunosuppression – may also be hirsuit because of the side-effects of cyclosporin. Look for scars (arteriovenous fistulae, transplanted organs), peritoneal dialysis catheters, central lines, pelvic masses (transplanted kidneys!), peripheral pulmonary stenosis (Alagille's syndrome)
- Nephrotic syndrome – presence of protein in the urine and peripheral oedema if at presentation or in relapse
- Rarely – interstitial pneumonitis, cystic fibrosis (treatment of allergic bronchopulmonary aspergillosis), inflammatory bowel disease, juvenile chronic arthritis, chronic active hepatitis

Cushing's syndrome

Most commonly due to a malignant carcinoma, benign adenoma or nodular hyperplasia, over half occurring before the age of 3 years. Eighty-five per cent occur before the age of 8 years. Above this age, the most likely diagnosis is Cushing's disease. Cushing's syndrome can rarely be caused by ectopic ACTH production, e.g. Wilm's tumour, phaeochromocytoma, neuroblastoma and pancreatic islet cell tumours.

Investigations

- FBC – polycythaemia, lymphopenia and eosinopenia.
- U&E's – hypokalaemia, hypochloraemia
- Blood gas – alkalosis
- Diurnal blood cortisol levels – loss of the normal diurnal variation (normal is highest at 08:00 h, falling to < 50% at 20:00 h in children over 3 years of age)
- Urinary 17-hydroxyprogesterone levels (↑)
- Dexamethasone suppression test
- Bone age (may be retarded, normal or advanced) and bone density measurement, e.g. DEXA scan, for osteoporosis
- MRI of the sella turcica

Cushing's disease

- Secondary to either microscopic or macroscopic pituitary adenomas
- Nelson's syndrome is a covert pituitary adenoma that presents itself only after bilateral adrenalectomy for Cushing's disease

N.B. Five endocrine causes for a short and fat child – Cushing's syndrome, hypothyroidism, hypopituitarism, growth hormone deficiency and pseudohypoparathyroidism.

Cystic fibrosis

Examine this boy's respiratory system

This very thin adolescent boy is peripherally and centrally cyanosed with *clubbing* of his fingers and toes. He has an abnormally shaped chest with *increased anterior-posterior diameter, Harrison's sulci* and *hyperinflation*. His resting respiratory rate is 23 breaths per minute and during the examination he demonstrated a productive sounding *cough* and *halitosis*. Percussion note is resonant in all lung fields, but auscultation reveals only reasonable air entry throughout with bilateral *coarse crepitations* and *expiratory wheeze*. To complete my examination I would like to carry out 3 peak flow measurements, plot his height and weight on the appropriate centile chart, dipstick his urine (to exclude glycosuria [corticosteroids, diabetes mellitus]) and look in the sputum pot by the side of his bed. My working diagnosis is *cystic fibrosis*.

Notes

- Autosomal recessive
- 1 in 22 carriers in the white population of the UK, incidence 1 in 2500
- Chromosome 7, 70% of UK caucasians are ΔF508 homozygotes
- Genetic mutations result in a defective cystic fibrosis trans–membrane conductance regulator that is found on the surface of epithelial cells and acts as a 'gateway' for chloride to leave the cell
- Neonatal screening, using the Guthrie card to measure serum immunoreactive trypsin (IRT) is undertaken in some centres within the UK (only 22% of newborn babies covered by this screening programme). If the IRT is elevated, the genetic mutations resulting in CF can be looked for on the original Guthrie card blood spot. The benefit of earlier diagnosis by means of neonatal screening remains contentious
- Median age of survival is ~31 years if born with CF in 1998 (median survival of 2 years in 1960)
- Males are infertile, women are sub-fertile with a pregnancy rate of ~ 4% per year (17 to 37-year-olds). Pregnancy results in a significant fall in respiratory function that is often not recoverable

X-rays

The Crispin Norman and Northern paediatric respiratory scores are measures of disease severity based on chest X-ray findings. These include bronchial wall thickening, cystic changes, areas of collapse and consolidation and bronchiectatic changes. The Schwachmann score encompasses weight, height, clinical and chest X-ray findings to measure disease severity.

Differential diagnosis

- Kartagener's syndrome (see page 86)
- Primary ciliary dyskinesia
- Inhalation of a foreign body (localised bronchiectasis)
- Post-infective bronchiectasis, e.g. tuberculosis, whooping cough, measles (localised or generalised)
- Williams–Campbell syndrome
- Congenital cystic bronchiectasis

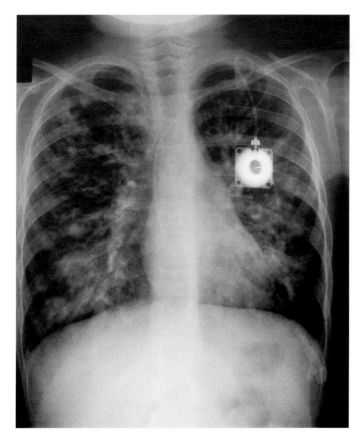

Fig. 13 Typical X-ray changes seen in CF (Portacath in situ)

Cystic hygroma (lymphangioma)

Examine this boy's neck

On inspection this young boy has a large *swelling* arising from his parotid region. There is no overlying erythema or skin change. On palpation the mass is soft and compressible and appears fluid filled. It *transilluminates* and there is no bruit or palpable thrill. It is non-tender. I think that this boy has a *cystic hygroma*.

Notes

- Aetiology
  - developmental defect in lymphatic pathways
  - failure of embryonic lymph sacs to communicate with the venous system
- Benign abnormal collections of lymphatic vessels
- May be single or multicystic and can be extensive
- Contain straw–coloured fluid
- Most arise in the posterior triangle of the neck but they may affect the tongue or root of upper limbs
- 60% present at birth
  - may be diagnosed antenatally
  - may obstruct labour
- 90% present by end of second year
- 10% have intrathoracic extension – 'amoebic' like spread results in intimate connections to trachea and other structures of the neck
- May compromise airway and interfere with swallowing – tracheostomy may be required

Treatment

- Surgical excision
- Adjunctive therapies
  - intralesional bleomycin injections
  - intralesional OK-432 (strain of *Streptococcus pyogenes*)
  - percutaneous embolisation

If small amounts of cystic tumour are left the recurrence risk is 10–15%.

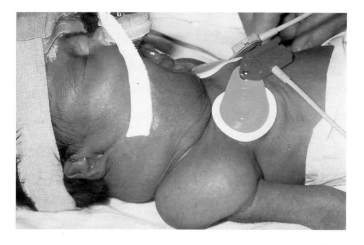

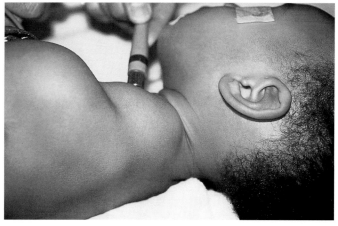

Figs 14 & 15 Note attempt at transillumination

Dermatomyositis

What do you think about this girl's limbs?

This 12-year-old *Cushingoid* girl is in a wheelchair and requires support to transfer to the bed. She cannot walk unaided but can move all four limbs against gravity (power 4/5). Muscle mass is poor and passive movements are uncomfortable. Tone, sensation, co-ordination and reflexes are normal. During the examination I have noticed a purple discolouration to the upper eyelids (pathognomic *heliotrope rash*), erythematous lesions in a butterfly distribution on the face and scaly erythema over the extensor surfaces of several joints, particularly the inter-phalangeal joints (*Göttron's papules*). She has no difficulty swallowing her own secretions or a drink of water and she has no cardio-respiratory distress. This child has *dermatomyositis* and has been treated with corticosteroids.

Notes

- Unusual before age 2 years, peak onset in childhood between 5 and 15 years
- Females more commonly affected than males. Familial cases have been reported
- Unknown aetiology
  - immunological
  - infection (Coxsackie, Mycobacteria, Staphylococcus)
  - genetic predisposition (HLA-B8)
  - immunisations and medications have been incriminated

Features

- Generalised malaise – low grade pyrexia, fatigue, misery, insidious onset
- Muscle weakness – *proximal > distal, generalised* and *symmetrical*
- Skin – peri-orbital *heliotrope rash*, facial oedema, *Göttron's papules* that later become hypo- or hyper-pigmented, peri-ungual telangectasia
- Miscellaneous – dysphagia, small bowel dysmotility, dysphonia, diplopia

The muscle weakness demonstrated may in part be due to the corticosteroids. Look for other evidence of corticosteroid administration with 'buffalo hump', abdominal striae and thinning of the skin (see page 78).

In adults dermatomyositis is associated with malignancy, but this is rarely the case in children (isolated case reports only).

Investigations

- Elevated muscle enzymes – creatine phosphokinase and aldolase are the most useful
- ESR/plasma viscosity
- Electromyography – can be normal in 10% of children
- Muscle biopsy – may be normal
- X-rays – calcinosis of the muscle around joints. Computerised tomography may demonstrate calcinosis earlier than plain X-ray

Differential diagnosis

- Other connective tissue disorders – SLE, JCA (see page 134), scleroderma, sarcoidosis
- Neuro-muscular disease – Guillain–Barré syndrome (see page 108), polio (asymmetrical), myasthenia gravis
- Trichinosis – *Trichinella spiralis* larval ingestion from infected meat. Adult worms mature in the gut and migrate to striated muscle producing myalgia and peri-orbital oedema. Elevated IgE together with a history of eating uncooked meat

Prognosis

The disease has two stages, an early, inflammatory phase (lasting 1–2 years) and a chronic phase. Calcinosis of the muscles is a marker of the end of the inflammatory phase and occurs frequently in children (~65%).

- Contractures are common
- Gastrointestinal perforation due to the vasculitis may occur and should be suspected in a child with dermatomyositis who suddenly becomes unwell. Corticosteroids may mask the symptoms of perforation
- Hyperandrogenism, insulin resistance and lipodystrophy are described as late complications
- Mortality is < 10% if treated. Death occurs as a result of involvement of palato-respiratory musculature
- Around 50% of survivors will have significant sequelae

Dextrocardia

Examine this young boy's cardiovascular system

On general inspection this boy is not cyanosed and has no respiratory distress although I note that he has *nasal polyps* and a *productive sounding cough*. His chest shape is normal and there are no scars. Examination of his hands reveals *finger clubbing* but no splinter haemorrhages or cyanosis. His pulse is of normal rate, rhythm, character and volume. The femoral pulses are normal. His apex beat is located in the 5th right intercostal space. There are no thrills or heaves and heart sounds are normal. I would like to measure his blood pressure, examine his respiratory and abdominal system and perform a chest X-ray to confirm the position of the cardiac shadow.

This young boy has *dextrocardia* and *finger clubbing*. The most likely diagnosis is Kartagener's syndrome.

Notes

Kartagener's syndrome
- autosomal recessive
- 1 in 32 000 live births
- accounts for 50% of cases of primary ciliary dyskinesia (PCD)

Features
- Situs inversus
- Chronic nasal discharge
- Sinusitis
- Bronchiectasis
- Male infertility
- Females may be subfertile

Differential diagnosis

- Cystic fibrosis
- Immunodeficiency
- α1-antitrypsin deficiency
- TB

Diagnosis

Saccharin test
A saccharin tablet is placed on the nasal turbinate and the time taken for it to be tasted is recorded. Normal 12–15 minutes. Prolonged with PCD.

Nasal brushings
Examine under high magnification interference light microscopy and electron microscopy.

Management

- Physiotherapy
- Antibiotics for respiratory symptoms
- Immunoprophylaxis – influenza vaccination

Prognosis

- Life expectancy normal with good treatment

Down's syndrome

Comment on this girl's appearance

This *short* girl has *brachycephaly, slanting palpebral fissures, low set ears with a flattened upper helix, bilateral epicanthic folds, depressed nasal bridge* and *a protruding tongue.* She is centrally cyanosed and I would like to examine her cardiovascular system for evidence of cyanotic heart disease. She has *broad spade-like hands* with *clindodactyly* and a *single palmar crease* (simian crease). She has a gap between her 1st and 2nd toe (ape-line). Her features are consistent with *Down's syndrome* with associated *congenital heart disease.*

Genetics

1. Non-dysjunction (95%)
   - 47XX, + 21 or 47XY, +21
   - Usually arises due to non-dysjunction in maternal meiosis
   - Incidence increases with maternal age
2. Translocation (3%)
   - Most commonly a Robertsonian 14, 21 translocation giving a karyotype in an affected child of 45XX, −14, + t (14q21q)
   - Translocations involving chromosome 22, 15, 13, 21 also seen
   - Inheritance of one normal chromosome 21 from each parent plus a translocation chromosome involving chromosome 21. Carrier parent is phenotypically normal despite having one normal 21 chromosome, one normal 14 chromosome and a fused 21, 14 chromosome giving a karyotype of 45XX, −14, −21 (or 45XY, −14, −21). Female carrier of 14q21q or 13q21q Robertsonian translocation has a recurrence risk of 15% in further pregnancies, male carriers a 3–5% risk
3. Mosaic (2%) – can have normal IQ

Notes

- Most common autosomal trisomy
- Natural prevalence 1:600 live births. Incidence in UK = 0.9 : 1000 live births

Newborn
- Hypotonia
- Poor feeding
- Umbilical hernia
- Excess skin at back of neck

Cardiovascular
- Congenital heart disease seen in 50%
- Atrio-ventricular septal defects most common
- Fallot's, ASD's, VSD's seen

Ophthalmology
- Brushfield spots, refractive errors in 70%
- Congenital cataracts, strabismus, glaucoma, nystagmus also seen

Orthopaedic
- Atlantoaxial subluxation (ligamentous laxity of C1)
- Pes planus, metatarsus varus, scoliosis, patellar instability, subluxation/dislocation of hips

ENT
- Hearing loss in 50% (conductive most common)
- Upper airway obstruction, obstructive sleep apnoea and persistent mucopurulent nasal discharge
- High arched palate
- Irregular dentition

Endocrinology
- Short stature. Specific growth charts exist
- Males and females subfertile
- Hyper/hypothyroidism

Gastroenterology
- 10% have congenital malformations – atresias of jejunum, duodenum, oesophagus and anus
- Annular pancreas, exomphalos, coeliac disease (4%), Hirschsprung's disease (2%), gastro-intestinal reflux also seen

Haematology
- Leukaemia (1st year of life – acute non-lymphoblastic; older children – acute lymphoblastic)

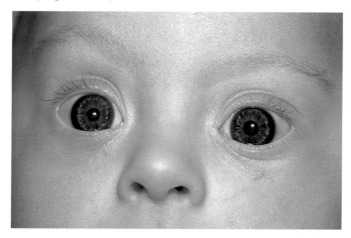

Fig. 16   Brushfield spots in Down's syndrome

Immunology
- Immunodeficiency – cell-mediated
- Autoimmune disease – hypothyroidism (seen in 10%), hyperthyroidism, autoimmune chronic active hepatitis, primary sclerosing cholangitis, IDDM, Addison's disease, alopecia, vitiligo

Dermatology
- Dry skin
- Folliculitis

Neurology
- Infantile spasms
- Autism
- Depression
- IQ: 25–75
- Early onset Alzheimer's disease

Hands
- Single palmar crease – 50% (Simian crease, seen in 2–3% of normal people)
- Abnormal dermatoglyphics (high axial triradius)
- Low set thumb
- Bridged palmar line (Sydney line)
- Hypoplasia of middle phalanx of fifth finger

Duchenne muscular dystrophy

Examine this boy's gait

Christopher is a 6-year-old boy with a '*waddling*' (classical description but may be deemed as offensive by parents!) *lordotic* (due to weakness of the extensor muscles of the spine) gait. He has a *positive Trendelenberg sign* (the pelvis tilts downwards on the opposite side when standing on one leg – a sign of gluteal muscle weakness in DMD). He is not particularly safe on his feet and tends to fall forwards. Running exaggerates his tendency to *toe-walk*. When asked to stand up from lying, he demonstrates a positive *Gower's sign*. Examining his legs in more detail he has wasted thigh muscles and bulky calves (*pseudo-hypertrophy*) and limited dorsi-flexion at the ankles (occurs from shortening of the Achilles tendon and causes toe-walking as the child gets older). Tone, sensation and co-ordination are normal but reflexes are absent at the knee and ankle (may be preserved until late). His plantar reflexes are down-going. I think this boy has *Duchenne muscular dystrophy*.

Notes

- Incidence = 1 : 3000–4000 male births
- X-linked recessive, but 30% are new mutations
- Due to absence of dystrophin, a protein of the sarcolemal membrane of muscle
- To demonstrate the Gower's sign properly, start with the child lying supine. A child without DMD would simply sit up and then stand, whereas a child with DMD has to turn himself prone before attempting to stand and 'climb up himself'
- The presenting complaint in DMD is often speech delay and the child not walking properly or his walking becoming abnormal/clumsy
- Around one-third of children have moderate developmental delay. All have a degree of intellectual impairment
- Urinary and bowel continence are maintained until late in the illness
- Progressive generalised scoliosis occurs with increasing weakness and loss of independent mobility

Investigations

- Creatinine phosphokinase (CPK) – should be used as a screening test for all boys not walking by 18 months of age or with a deterioration of gait at any age. CPK is elevated into the tens of thousands but falls with disease progression (as muscle mass diminishes). Asymptomatic female carriers will demonstrate elevated CPK levels in ~80% of cases

- EMG – myopathic changes
- Genetic analysis – for known chromosome Xp21 deletions
- Muscle biopsy – absence of dystrophin, presence of adipose and fibrous connective tissue. This investigation may now be out-dated with genetic advancements but if in doubt it must be done
- ECG – cardiomyopathic changes
- Death usually occurs by late teens from cardiorespiratory failure
- DMD has been seen in girls with Turner's syndrome because they have only one X chromosome that carries the Xp21 deletion for DMD

Differential diagnosis

1. Becker muscular dystrophy
   Less common with very similar clinical and investigative findings. However, developmental delay is unusual and disease progression is much slower. If a child is walking still at age 12, the child has Becker MD rather than DMD. Death occurs in the 3rd to 5th decade of life.
2. Inflammatory myopathies
   Coxsackie B myositis, dermatomyositis (see page 84). CPK can be hugely elevated but tends to be transient.
3. Spinal muscular atrophy
   Type III (Kugelberg–Welander disease). Usually autosomal recessive inheritance. Presents with problems walking at around age 2 years because of increasing weakness of the pelvic girdle causing a 'waddling' gait. Shoulder girdle weakness also occurs with 'winging' of the scapulae. Fasciculations of the tongue present. Diagnosis by EMG (fibrillation potentials), creatinine kinase ↑.

Ectodermal dysplasia

Describe Harry's hair

This 6-year-old boy (X-linked recessive) has very *sparse, fine, wispy scalp hair* and *absent eyelashes and eyebrows*. His *skin is pale, dry and smooth* (hairless). His nails are normal but dentition is markedly abnormal with only a couple of *cone-shaped ('peg') teeth*. He is *dysmorphic* because of *mid-facial hypoplasia* (as a result of defective dentition development), thickened dry lips and frontal bossing. I would like to examine his chest (externally for absent [*athelia*] or extra nipples [*polythelia*] and internally for recurrent bacterial infections), assess his swallowing (*dry mucous membranes*) and look at his eyes for the presence of *corneal opacities*.

I think he has *anhydrotic ectodermal dysplasia*.

Notes

- Anihidrotic ectodermal dysplasia is one of a group of conditions caused by abnormal development of tissues of ectodermal origin, i.e. hair, nails, teeth, sweat glands. Therefore if asked in the exam to examine a child's hair, always look at the nails, skin and teeth
- Inheritance for the other ectodermal dysplasias are autosomal recessive (associated brachydactyly), autosomal dominant (normal sweating, lichenified skin over bony prominences, normal facies and teeth, but dystrophic nails – **look for evidence of disease in accompanying parent**)
- The condition requires input and follow-up from the dentists, ophthalmologists, geneticists, paediatricians +/− surgeons. Advice regarding the avoidance of hot weather is essential

Eczema

Examine this boy's skin

This boy has an erythematous, dry itchy rash on the flexor surfaces of both arms. There are areas of hyperpigmentation and thickened dry skin (*lichenification*). There are numerous areas of *excoriation*. The diagnosis is *eczema*.

Notes

- Atopic eczema affects 3–5% of children < 5 years old
- Family history of atopy seen in 70%
- 40% of children with atopic eczema will develop asthma/hay fever
- Aetiology is unknown

Infantile eczema

- Onset 2–6 months old
- Affects – forehead, face and extensor surfaces
- Clinical
  - dry/wet, oozing, crusting
  - erythematous
  - papules and vesicles
  - intense pruritus – excoriation marks

Childhood eczema

- Onset 4–10 years old
- Affects – popliteal and antecubital fossae, ankles, wrists
- Clinical
  - dry/wet
  - erythematous
  - chronic dry and thickened – lichenification
  - pruritus

Complications

- Secondary infection
  - bacterial (*Staphylococcus aureus*, β haemolytic *Streptococcus*)
  - viral (herpes)

Treatment

- Emollient – aqueous cream to prevent drying

- Avoidance of perfumed soaps, biological washing powders
- Bath oil
- Decrease itching
  - short fingernails
  - cotton mittens
  - night sedation
- Topical/systemic antibiotics
- Topical corticosteroids

Ehlers–Danlos syndrome

What do you notice about this 3-year-old boy?

Initial inspection reveals *scarring* of his skin overlying bony prominences, particularly his knees. His skin is rather thin and there are several large *ecchymoses*. Pulling the skin over his elbow he demonstrates marked skin *hyperelasticity*. I am able to extend his elbows and knees beyond normal full extension, suggesting a degree of *joint laxity* (if cooperative and in older children get them to pull their thumb back to see if they can touch the flexor aspect of their forearm). His hair and teeth are normal and he has normal sclerae. I would like to undertake fundoscopy to exclude retinal problems (detachment and perforation, seen in type VI) and examine his cardiovascular system (valvular regurgitation). This boy has *Ehlers–Danlos syndrome*.

Notes

- Ehlers–Danlos syndrome is a connective tissue disorder due to (presumed, in some cases) defective collagen or procollagen. Inheritance is varied and signs and symptoms dependent upon type
- Affected individuals are normal at birth
- The most likely examples seen in the part II examination are going to demonstrate hyperelastic skin, with bruising, fragility and poor healing and joint laxity
- Associated features include herniae, heart valve incompetences, alopecia, contractures, pes planus and blue sclerae

Classifications

For completeness, the classification is included (but realistically cannot be expected!!).

- Type I – Autosomal dominant (AD). Hyperextensible, soft skin with easy bruising and dystrophic scarring, hyperextensible joints. Associated prematurity (PROM)
- Type II – AD. Milder form than type I
- Type III – AD. Joint hypermobility. Skin manifestations are milder
- Type IV – AD and autosomal recessive (AR). Severe bruising, thin skin, prominent veins
- Type V – X-linked. Marked skin hyperelasticity but mild scarring, fragility and bruising

- Type VI – AR. Eye involvement. Retinal perforation and detachment. Scoliosis
- Type VII – AD and AR. Arthrochalasis multiplex congenita
- Type VIII – AD. Periodontitis type – premature loss of teeth. Marfanoid habitus
- Type IX – X-linked recessive. 'Occipital horn syndrome'. Low serum copper and caeruloplasmin
- Type X – AR. Fibronectin abnormality – failure of platelet aggregation

Differential diagnosis

- Cutis laxa – AR and AD inheritance
  - Premature ageing appearance of newborn babies ('bloodhound' appearance). The skin hangs down rather than being hyperextensible

Treatment

- None
- Arterial rupture may result in premature death, particularly type IV

Epidermolysis bullosa

Examine this boy's skin. What do you think the diagnosis is?

This young boy has numerous *scars* over both knees. I note that he also has a few *blisters* on his right knee. His hair appears normal. His nails are *dysplastic*. The most likely diagnosis is *epidermolysis bullosa*.

Notes

Three major groups:

1. Junctional epidermolysis bullosa
   - Autosomal recessive
   - Split between basal cell and basal lamina
   - Onset at birth
   - Heals with no scarring
   - Mucosal, involvement
   - Dysplastic nails, teeth
2. Epidermolysis bullosa simplex
   - Autosomal dominant
   - Split is supra-basal
   - Onset when children become mobile
   - Heals with no scarring
   - No mucosal involvement
   - Normal nails, hair, teeth
3. Dystrophic epidermolysis bullosa
   Two forms:
   - Autosomal dominant
     - mild disease
     - blister – heals with scars
     - hair, teeth normal
   - Autosomal recessive
     - severe disease
     - large blisters present at birth – heals with scars
     - formation of webs between fingers/toes
     - hair, teeth, nails, mucous membranes abnormal
     - ↑ risk of squamous cell carcinoma in scars

Erythema nodosum

Look at this girl's legs

This 14-year-old girl complains of *painful shins*. On examination she has several areas of *erythematous* change overlying both tibiae. The areas are slightly *raised*, varying in diameter with *indistinct margins* and have a *shiny* appearance. They are *tender* to touch (**be careful not to hurt the patient!**) and are warmer than the surrounding normal looking skin. She does not have the rash in other areas (although it can occasionally be seen on the thighs, buttocks and upper limbs). She has *erythema nodosum*. Although in 50% of cases no cause is found, I would look at the throat for evidence of a bacterial pharyngitis and in the mouth and perineum for evidence of inflammatory bowel disease.

Notes

- Causes:
  - idiopathic – 50% of cases
  - group A β-haemolytic Streptococci
  - drugs – sulphonamide antibiotics, oral contraceptive pill
  - tuberculosis
  - inflammatory bowel disease
  - viral – Ebstein–Barr, hepatitis
  - miscellaneous – Behçet's disease, SLE, sarcoidosis, fugal infections, cat-scratch fever
- A vasculitic process of unknown aetiology
- Worthwhile investigations include a throat swab, ESR and anti-streptolysin O titres
- Treatment with non-steroidal anti-inflammatory drugs or oral corticosteroids rarely

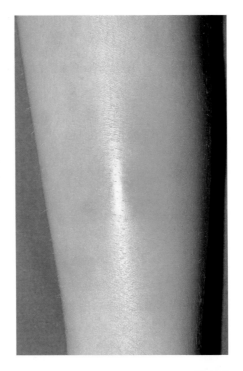

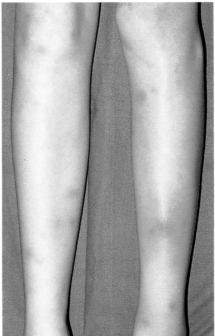

Figs 17 & 18   Erythema nodosum

Fallot's tetralogy

Examine this child's cardiovascular system

This 18-month-old is centrally and peripherally *cyanosed* at rest in air. He has the phenotypic appearance of *Down's syndrome* (see page 88) (offer to plot his length/height on the appropriate centile chart). General inspection reveals a left-sided *thoractomy scar* and, in conjunction with an absent radial pulse on this side, I suspect he has had a *Blalock–Taussig shunt* (anastomosis between a subclavian artery and a pulmonary artery to increase blood flow to the lungs). He is not tachypnoeic (measure the rate) or dyspnoeic but does have *clubbing* of his fingers, thumb and toes. His apex beat is not displaced (mid-clavicular line, 4th/5th intercostal space), but there is a lower left para-sternal thrill (*right ventricular hypertrophy*) and a thrill in the pulmonary area (left, 2nd intercostal space, due to *pulmonary stenosis*). Auscultation reveals a *single 2nd heart sound* and an *ejection systolic murmur* in the pulmonary area that does not radiate to the neck, consistent with *pulmonary stenosis*. There is also a *continuous soft murmur* heard loudest over the left upper anterior chest consistent with a *shunt murmur*. The chest is clear. He does not have hepatomegaly and femoral pulses are present. I would like to go on and measure four limb blood pressure using an appropriately sized blood pressure cuff.

This boy has complex *cyanotic congenital heart disease* together with *Down's syndrome*. The presence of *pulmonary stenosis* and *cyanosis* gives the possibility of *Fallot's tetralogy* – to confirm this I would like a chest X-ray and ECG (say this provided you know what to look for from these investigations!).

Notes

- Pulmonary stenosis, over-riding aorta, ventricular septal defect and right ventricular hypertrophy = *Fallot's tetralogy*
- Plot height and weight on the appropriate centile chart to assess whether the child is failing to thrive – this may suggest that earlier corrective surgery is necessary
- ECG – right atrial hypertrophy (peaked P wave), right ventricular hypertrophy (R > S in V_1, right axis deviation, +ve T wave in V_1)
- CXR – boot-shaped heart, decreased pulmonary vasculature, 25% have a right-sided aortic arch

Complications of tetralogy

- 'Hyper-cyanotic' episodes, due to spasm of the right ventricular infundibulum
- Treatment with knees to chest position, oxygen, morphine and corrective surgery
- Thrombotic stroke – hemiplegia
- Cerebral abscess
- Bacterial endocarditis

N.B. For older child check for the state of the teeth and warn parents about the need for prophylactic antibiotics.

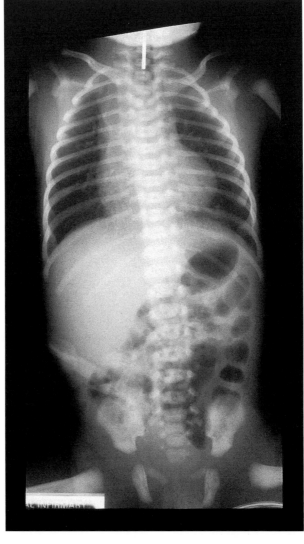

Fig. 19 'Boot'-shaped heart and oligamic lung fields. Note oesophageal atresia

Floppy infant

Examine this boy

This 3-month-old boy on first inspection appears alert, interested in his surroundings and responds to my voice. He has supplemental oxygen via nasal prongs and has a naso-gastric tube in situ. Prone he adopts the '*frog-leg*' position (external rotation of the hips and flexion of the knees) and he is unable to lift his head off the bed. On ventral suspension he appears generally *floppy* (rag doll). Supine he has a *paucity of spontaneous movement* with *significant head lag* on pulling to sit. On vertical suspension attempted weight bearing is minimal. Muscle tone is generally reduced and I am unable to elicit any of the tendon reflexes. I note a see-saw pattern of breathing (*diaphragmatic breathing*) and *fasciculation of the tongue*. These findings are consistent with a diagnosis of *Werdnig–Hoffmann (type I) spinal muscular atrophy*.

Notes

- Incidence = 1 : 25 000
- Autosomal recessive inheritance
- 50% present at birth with generalised weakness, hypotonia, joint deformity and respiratory difficulty. A history of reduced fetal movements towards the end of pregnancy can sometimes be elicited. The rest present before 6 months of age with failure to thrive, poor feeding, generalised weakness and floppiness. Recurrent chestiness/pneumonias occur because of a weak cough and chronic aspiration. The infant appears alert because of sparing of the facial muscles
- 95% die within 18 months from respiratory failure and pneumonia

Differential diagnosis

It is essential to differentiate between 'central' and 'peripheral' causes for hypotonia. As a general rule babies with central causes do not have significant muscle weakness and the reflexes are easily elicited. Hypotonia, weakness, absent reflexes and normal development are suggestive of a peripheral causation.

Central
- Chromosomal/genetic disorders
- Down's syndrome
- Prader–Willi syndrome
- Lesch–Nyhan syndrome

- Hypotonic/atonic cerebral palsy secondary to pre-, peri- or post-natal hypoxic ischaemic encephalopathy
- Drugs

Peripheral
- Anterior horn cell
  - Werdnig–Hoffmann spinal muscular atrophy
  - poliomyelitis
- Peripheral nerve
  - Guillain–Barré syndrome see page 108
  - hereditary motor and sensory neuropathy
  - Riley–Day syndrome
  - congenital hypomyelinating neuropathy
  - metachromatic leucodystrophy
  - Krabbe's disease
- Neuromuscular junction
  - congenital myasthenia gravis
  - infantile botulism
- Muscle
  - myotonic dystrophy
  - congenital muscular dystrophy
  - congenital myopathy
  - endocrine myopathies – hypo- and hyper-thyroidism
  - metabolic-storage disease – glycogenoses (Pompe's) cytochrome oxidase deficiency, carnitine deficiency

The most common causes for a floppy infant seen in the exam will be dysmorphic syndromes, Werdnig–Hoffmann SMA, 'hypotonic' cerebral palsy (CP), congenital myotonic dystrophy and neonatal myasthenia gravis.

An infant with Down's syndrome or Prader–Willi syndrome will have characteristic dysmorphic features.

An infant with CP may have microcephaly, dolicocephaly (ex-prematurity), hand fisting, increased tendon reflexes, lower limb scissoring, 'advanced' weight-bearing and developmental delay.

If myotonic dystrophy is suspected, ask mother to clench her fist and open her hand rapidly (better test than the classic textbook handshake test). Try and elicit a history of polyhydramnios (poor fetal swallowing), decreased fetal movements during pregnancy, prolonged labour and respiratory difficulties in the neonatal period. The infant will have an expressionless face with tenting of the mouth ('fish' mouth). Varying degrees of arthrogryposis may be present.

Myasthenia gravis (MG) would be suggested by an expressionless face with bilateral ptosis ± ophthalmoplegia, feeble cry and poor feeding. Neonatal MG occurs as a result of trans-placental passage of anti-acetylcholine receptor antibodies, is transient (4–6 weeks) and examination of the mother's face will help make the diagnosis. Congenital MG is an autosomal recessive condition and the mother may not have the disease.

Investigations

Anterior horn cell disease
- Electromyography
- In SMA-reduced interference pattern, long duration potentials and spontaneously discharging units
- Characteristic denervation or fibrillation potentials may be seen
- Muscle biopsy and creatinine kinase may be normal

Peripheral nerve disease
- Nerve conduction studies

Neuromuscular junction
- Edrophonium test
- For MG also perform mediastinal imaging (for a thymic shadow), acetylcholine antibody test and EMG (fatiguability)

Muscle disease
- Congenital myotonic dystrophy
  - elevated creatinine kinase
  - myopathic EMG (of baby and mother)
  - muscle biopsy demonstrating fibrous tissue and fat between muscle fibres

Fragile X syndrome (Martin–Bell syndrome)

> ## Comment on this boy's appearance
>
> This boy is *tall*, has a *large head, large jaw, large everted ears* and a *prominent broad forehead*. He is *developmentally delayed*. I would like to examine his joints for evidence of *hyper extensibility* and undertake a cardiovascular examination (prolapsed heart valves). My diagnosis is *Fragile X syndrome* although I would like to examine his testicles to confirm this.

Notes

- X-linked disorder
- Incidence = 1 : 1000 males (1 : 2000 females)
- Most common cause of inherited mental retardation (4–8% of all mentally retarded males) IQ < 50 in 25% of affected boys
- Epilepsy occasionally
- Behaviour
  - infants are shy and have gaze aversion
  - affected children are hyperactive and have a decreased attention span
  - echolalia (repetitive speech)

N.B. Other triplet diseases – Huntington's disease, dystrophia myotonica, X-linked bulbospinal neuronopathy

Features

- Macro-orchidism (testis > 25 ml) after puberty with normal testicular histology and testosterone synthesis
- Pes planus
- Obesity
- High-arched palate
- Pectus excavatum
- Connective tissue dysfunction (hernias)
- Prolapse of aortic and mitral valves

Genetics

Fragile site at Xq27.3 (near the telomere of the long arm of the X chromosome). This is seen in 5–50% of cells from an affected male. Culture medium used for chromosome analysis must be deficient in folate or thymidine. The Fragile X mental retardation gene (FMR-1) is a region containing a long CGG trinucleotide repeat sequence. In a normal person this repeat sequence is seen 6–54 times. The number of repeats is unstable and if the gene contains 60–200 repeats the patients are said to have a *premutation*. A male with a premutation will pass it to all his daughters. When these daughters have sons of their own there is a risk that the premutation undergoes *expansion* to greater than 200 repeats, resulting in Fragile X syndrome. Males and females with a premutation are of normal intelligence. Females with the full mutation may be normal (50%), or have mild (30%) or moderate (~1%) mental retardation.

Differential diagnosis

1. Soto's syndrome
   - Sporadic occurrence
   - Advanced bone maturation
   - Macrocephaly
   - Large hands and feet
   - Prominent forehead
   - Down-slanting palpebral fissures
   - Prognathism
   - Hypertelorism
   - Coarse facies
   - Fits
   - Poor co-ordination
   - Narrow anterior mandible
2. Laurence–Moon–Biedl syndrome – see page 183
3. Marfan's syndrome – see page 147

Guillain–Barré syndrome

Examine this young girl's lower limbs

On inspection she has no obvious abnormalities of her legs, in particular no wasting or fasciculation. She does, however, complain of some pain in her legs and they are tender on palpation. She has a *symmetrical flaccid paralysis* affecting both lower limbs. Her legs are *areflexic* and she has a *glove and stocking sensory loss*. I would like to perform a *peak flow* and examine her fully for any evidence of autonomic dysfunction.

The diagnosis is *Guillain–Barré syndrome*.

Notes

- Commonest peripheral neuropathy in children. Most common age 5–9 years old

Aetiology

- Unknown –Mycoplasma, Campylobacter jejuni
- Mild preceding febrile illness 10–28 days prior is common

Features

- Paralysis is ascending: legs → trunk → arms → bulbar muscles
- Glove and stocking sensory loss (severe limb pain sometimes seen)
- Meningism/papilloedema seen in 30% of cases
- Irritability
- Autonomic dysfunction
  - hypotension
  - hypertension
  - arrythmias
  - excessive sweating
  - flushing
  - peripheral vasoconstriction
  - urinary retention
  - disturbed gut function
- Maximum weakness seen usually within 10 days of onset of symptoms
- 15% need ventilation due to respiratory muscle involvement

Investigations

- CSF – ↑ protein (often normal in first week), normal cell count
- Nerve conduction velocity ↓↓
- EMG – may show acute denervation

Differential diagnosis

- Transverse myelitis, polymyositis, dermatomyositis
- Poliomyelitis

Management

- Symptomatic and supportive
- Respiratory function monitoring (PEFR, oxygen saturations)
- Blood gas analysis
- Physiotherapy
  - passive movement of paralysed limbs
  - prevention of contractures
  - postural chest drainage
  - decrease risk of DVT/PE
- Steroids – no longer recommended
- Plasma exchange
  - decreases the interval until recovery
  - best results if given within 2 weeks of onset
- IV immunoglobulin – as effective as plasma exchange

Mortality

- 5% (respiratory failure, cardiovascular collapse)

Prognosis

- 80% – full recovery (may take up to 3–30 months)
- 20% – varying degrees of permanent muscle weakness

Hemiplegia

What do you notice about this infant?

This 8-month-old boy is sitting unsupported on the floor, playing with a toy but using only one hand. He shows marked hand preference (certainly abnormal before 12 months of age) for the right side. Although there is some spontaneous movement of the left arm, it is not against gravity. The fist of his left side is clenched and the arm has adopted a typical upper limb *hemiplegic* posture (wrist and elbow flexion, ulnar deviation, adducted and internally rotated at the shoulder). On standing with support the left leg is held adducted, flexed at the knee and plantar-flexed at the ankle. Both the left leg and arm are wasted with decreased muscle mass compared to the right. Both limbs also feel cooler to the touch (vasomotor instability). Tone is increased on the left side and joint reflexes are brisk. Both plantar reflexes are up-going (until the child walks at which time the normal right side will become down-going) and the lateral parachute reflexes are asymmetrical (leave until last as this will upset the hemiplegic infant). I would like to perform an eye examination including visual fields (for *hemianopia*).

Notes

• In older children encourage them to get off the bed, walk, hop and run down the ward.

Causes

• Acute
  • idiopathic
  • vascular malformations – A–V malformation, arterial and venous aneurysms
  • arterial occlusions – arteritis, Moyamoya disease, hypertension, trauma (including NAI), arteriosclerosis
  • venous occlusions – venous thrombosis, e.g. Factor V leidin deficiency
  • cerebral disease – post-ictal, encephalitis, cerebral abscess, cerebral tumour, multiple sclerosis
  • migraine
• Chronic
  • congenital hemiplegia – porencephalic cysts, pre-natal cerebral infarcts, focal cerebral atrophy
  • any of the above with incomplete resolution

N.B. Fog's sign – whilst standing, ask the patient to roll their ankles out, i.e. external rotation. If a subtle hemiplegia is present the upper limb on the affected side may adopt the classical hemiplegic posture, where before it was not evident.

Henoch–Schönlein purpura (anaphylactoid purpura)

Examine this boy's legs

This boy has a *purpuric rash* affecting the extensor surface of both lower limbs and buttocks. In some areas the rash appears *urticarial*. The rash is *symmetrical* in nature. I note that he has a few purpuric spots on his trunk, over both elbows and on his face. He has bilateral swelling of his knees and ankles and is unable to weight bear. I would like to check a FBC (platelets), clotting screen, blood pressure and dipstick his urine looking for *haematuria*. The most likely diagnosis is *Henoch–Schönlein purpura*. I would also like to carry out an abdominal system examination looking for any evidence of gut involvement.

Notes

- Most common vasculitis in children – affects 15 : 100 000 children per year
- 2 males : 1 female
- Age 2–8 most common
- Peak incidence – winter
- Aetiology – unknown (URTI common especially Streptococcal infections)
- Pathology – inflammatory haemorrhagic reaction of capillaries, small arterioles and venules. Diffuse, self-limiting vasculitis of immune mechanism – skin lesions and renal glomeruli contain C3 and IgA immune complexes

Other features

- Abdominal pain
  - seen in > 50%
  - pain due to haemorrhage into the gut wall
  - melaena, bloody diarrhoea and intussusception seen
- Arthritis
  - seen in 65%
  - pain and swelling in one or more joints (ankles and knees)
- Renal
  - haematuria, proteinuria, nephrotic/nephritic picture, hypertension
  - end-stage renal failure seen in 5–15%

- CNS
  - headache, fits, behavioural disturbances

Investigations

- Platelets, coagulation – normal
- ASOT

Treatment

- Symptomatic – monitor BP, urinalysis
- Analgesia for arthritis
- Severe abdominal pain – oral steroids

Prognosis

- 90% have self-limiting illness, most settling within 2–6 weeks
- Microscopic haematuria can occur for months or years
- Relapses can occur for up to 1 year
- Acute nephritis/nephrosis need long-term follow-up and all should have at least an annual blood pressure measurement

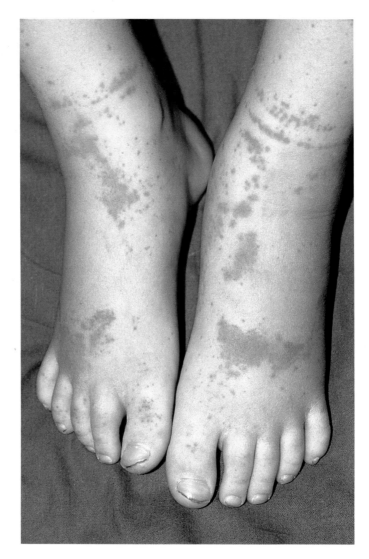

Fig. 20 Henoch–Schönlein purpura

Hepatomegaly

Examine this boy's abdomen

This boy is *jaundiced*. On inspection of his abdomen, there appears to be a mass in the right hypochondrium. Palpation reveals a mass arising from below the right costal margin which has a smooth, firm edge and extends 6 cm towards the right iliac fossa. I am unable to get above the mass and it moves downwards with respiration. The mass is dull to percussion. There is no evidence of splenomegaly and I would like to look for evidence of chronic liver disease including *spider naevi, palmar erythema, jaundice* and *pruritus*. The positive finding is that of *hepatomegaly*.

Notes

Aetiology
1. Infection
   - Bacterial (septicaemia)
   - Viral (hepatitis A, B, C, D, infectious mononucleosis, CMV, HIV)
   - Protozoal (malaria, toxoplasmosis)
   - Parasitic (hydatid)
2. Haematological
   - Sickle cell disease
   - Thalassaemia
3. Cardiovascular
   - Congestive cardiac failure
   - Constrictive pericarditis
   - IVC obstruction
4. Neoplastic
   - Leukaemia
   - Lymphoma
   - Hepatic tumours
   - Neuroblastoma
5. Metabolic
   - Galactossaemia
   - Glycogen storage disease
   - Wilson's disease
   - Urea cycle disorders
   - Storage disorders
   - α1-antitrypsin disease
6. Chronic disease
   - Still's disease

- Crohn's disease
- Ulcerative colitis
- SLE
- Cystic fibrosis
7. Portal hypertension

Hepatosplenomegaly

Examine this girl's abdomen

On inspection, this girl's abdomen appears full. On palpation, I can feel two masses, one in the right hypochondrium and one in the left hypochondrium. The mass in the right hypochondrium is present 7 cm below the costal margin. It has a smooth edge and moves down with respiration. I am unable to get above the mass and it is dull to percussion. The mass in the left hypochondrium extends towards the right iliac fossa. It moves down with respiration, is dull to percussion, has a notch on its medial aspect and I am unable to get above it. Both masses are non-tender. The diagnosis is *hepatosplenomegaly*.

Notes

Aetiology
1. Infection
   - Septicaemia
   - Hepatitis A, B
   - Infectious mononucleosis
2. Haematology
   - Sickle cell disease
   - Thalassaemia
   - Severe Fe deficiency anaemia
   - Hereditary spherocytosis
3. Neoplastic
   - Leukaemia
   - Lymphoma
4. Portal hypertension
5. Polycystic liver disease
6. Storage disorders

Hereditary spherocytosis

Examine this girl's abdominal system

On general inspection this 8-year-old caucasian girl has jaundice demonstrated by the discolouration of her sclera. Examination of her abdominal system reveals a mass in the left upper quadrant that is smooth and non-tender. Because I cannot get above this mass, it is dull to percussion and has a palpable notch, this is likely to be the spleen. Putting the *jaundice* and *splenomegaly* together, I think this child may have *hereditary spherocytosis*. A positive family history of intermittent *jaundice* and *splenomegaly* would obviously make this diagnosis even more probable. The presence of spherocytes on the blood film and a positive osmotic fragility test would be confirmatory evidence for the diagnosis.

Notes

- Autosomal recessive disorder
- 25% as a result of spontaneous mutation
- Investigation reveals a Coombs'-negative haemolysis with moderate anaemia and reticulocytosis
- N.B. Risk of splenic rupture secondary to trauma. If splenectomy has been performed, children should be on prophylactic penicillin.

Other causes of jaundice in well children

Inherited conjugated hyperbilirubinaemias are autosomal recessively inherited. Jaundice is mild and usually presents in adolescence or adulthood. It may only be apparent during infections, pregnancy, peri-operatively, during fasting or in subjects on the oral contraceptive pill. They are benign conditions and do not require treatment

- Dubin–Johnson syndrome
- Rotor syndrome

There are four broad categories for splenomegaly

- Haematological
  - HS
  - sickle cell disease (before 5 years of age)
  - haemolytic anaemia
  - thalassaemia
- Infection
  - bacterial – septicaemia, endocarditis, TB, brucella

- viral – infectious mononucleosis, hepatitis
- protozoa – malaria, leishmaniasis
- parasitic – schistosomiasis, hydatid disease
- Infiltration
  - leukemia
  - lymphoma
- Miscellaneous
  - connective tissue disorders – SLE, Felty's disease
  - storage disorders – Gaucher's, Niemann–Pick
  - amyloid, sarcoid, portal hypertension

See page 131 for discussion on jaundice.

Holt–Oram syndrome

Examine this boy's hands

This infant has *asymmetrical abnormalities of both upper limbs*. On the left side there is thumb hypoplasia only and on the right there is marked shortening of the distal limb, syndactyly and a triphalangeal thumb. Both shoulder girdles appear intact with full range of movement and clavicles can be palpated. I would like to X-ray the limbs and chest to identify the bony abnormalities and undertake a full cardiovascular examination. The association between *upper limb abnormalities* and *heart defects* is described as the *Holt–Oram syndrome*.

Notes

- Autosomal dominant
- Chromosome 14 or 12

Features

- Cardiac (85%) – ASD and VSD commonly, other defects in one-third including conduction defects
- Skeletal – thumb hypoplasia to phocomelia. Defects of the clavicle, scapula and sternum are associated. Asymmetrical limb defects are common
- Other – pectus excavatum, thoracic scoliosis, vertebral abnormalities, hypertelorism

Differential diagnosis

Congenital upper limb anomalies

- TAR syndrome – <u>T</u>hrombocytopenia, <u>A</u>bsent <u>R</u>adius see page 165
- Poland syndrome (see page 167)
- Klippel–Feil syndrome (cervical synostosis)
  - low hair line
  - short neck
  - genito-urinary abnormalities – horse-shoe kidney, renal, vaginal and ovarian agenesis
  - cardiovascular abnormalities – VSD, PDA, coarctation
  - neurological abnormalities – facial nerve palsy, ptosis, deafness
  - orthopaedic abnormalities – kyphoscoliosis, torticollis, Sprengel deformity, Poland syndrome, hemivertebrae

- Fanconi's pancytopenia
- Edward's syndrome (trisomy 18)
- Laurence–Moon–Biedl syndrome (see page 183)
- Meckel–Gruber syndrome
  - autosomal recessive
  - chromosome 17
  - occipital encephalocele
  - microcephaly
  - cleft lip and palate
  - post-axial polydactyly
  - congenital heart disease
  - ambiguous genitalia

Horner's syndrome

Examine this boy's face

This 2-year-old has *partial ptosis* of the left eye. Pupillary size is smaller on the left compared to the right but it is reactive to light and accommodation. Looking from above there is *enophthalmus* of the same eye. Although not detectable at the present time, *anhydrosis* may be found if the point of interruption to the sympathetic supply to the face and eye is proximal to the cervical ganglion. This child has a left-sided *Horner's syndrome*.

I note also that the boy is *cyanosed* at rest. I would like to examine his chest and neck for evidence of a scar (cyanotic heart disease that has required cardiac surgery).

Notes

• The triad of miosis, partial ptosis and enophthalmia make up Horner's syndrome

Causes and associations

• Klumpke's nerve palsy (C7, C8, T1) and associated cervical sympathetic chain injury
• Look for evidence of wasting of the small muscles of the hand
• Post-operative – cardiac, neck or thoracic surgery
• Neuroblastoma – ↑ urinary catecholamine excretion
• Vertebral anomalies
• Idiopathic
• Familial

Hurler's syndrome

What do Harriet's facial appearances make you think of?

She has very *coarse facies*, frontal bossing and I suspect *macrocephaly*, although I need to measure her OFC and plot it on the centile chart. She has *prominent lips*, a *short nose* and a *depressed nasal bridge*. She does not appear to fix on my face and there is a hazy appearance to the cornea, suggesting the presence of *cataracts*. She is wearing *bilateral hearing aids*. Looking more widely she has a *gibbus* and *kyphosis* of her lumbar spine, *short stature* and she has profound *developmental delay*. She demonstrates a '*claw-hand*' deformity with proximal tapering of the metacarpals and joint stiffness. Examining her abdomen, it is rather protuberant and I can detect *non-tender hepatomegaly* (x cm) and *splenomegaly* (x cm). There is an *umbilical hernia* but no inguinal herniae. The findings are compatible with a mucopolysaccharide disorder, the most likely being *Hurler's syndrome*.

Notes

The mucopolysaccharidoses arise because of defective metabolism of glycosaminoglycans (dermatan, keratan and heparan sulphates). All are autosomal recessive except Hunter's syndrome (X-linked recessive).

Hurler's syndrome

- Chromosome 4 (not chromosome 22 as reported in some texts)
- Defective enzyme is α–L–iduronidase
- Babies have normal physical features and radiological appearances at birth (although tissue accumulation of glycosaminoglycans can be detected)
- From around 3 months of age the infants develop rhinitis, recurrent infections and sometimes inguinal herniae
- From 6 months the features start to coarsen and the spinal abnormalities (dysostosis multiplex) develop
- Diagnosis is usual by about 9 months
- Death occurs before 10 years of age from congestive cardiac failure and respiratory infections

Scheie's syndrome

- Chromosome 4
- α–L–iduronidase defect also
- Normal stature and survival into adult life
- Corneal clouding is severe

Hunter's syndrome

- X-linked
- Defective enzyme is iduronate sulphatase
- Severe forms mimic Hurler's except for the absence of corneal clouding
- Milder forms occur and normal intelligence and life expectancy result

Sanfilippo syndrome

- Chromosome 17 and 12
- Insidious onset of intellectual deterioration and behavioural changes (including self-mutilation)
- Corneal clouding, hepatosplenomegaly and growth problems may be absent
- Mitral valve thickening can be severe

Morquio's disease

- Chromosome 3 and 16
- β-galactosidase and *N*-acetyl-galactosamine-6-sulphatase deficiencies respectively
- Severe skeletal abnormalities, cloudy cornea and aortic regurgitation
- Presentation in the first 2 years of life with genu valgum

Maroteaux–Lamy syndrome

- Chromosome 5
- Similar physical characteristics to Hurler's but developmental delay is rare
- Odontoid hypoplasia and cardiac involvement are frequent findings

Sly's syndrome

- Chromosome 7
- β-glucuronidase deficiency
- Very variable severity

Diagnosis

- Radiological abnormalities – dysostosis multiplex
- Urine analysis for ↑ glycosaminoglycan excretion
- Cultured fibroblast/leucocyte enzyme studies

Treatment

- Essentially supportive
- Bone marrow transplantation has been carried out in Hurler's syndrome, but its value is unproven

Ichthyoses

> **Examine this boy's skin**
>
> This young boy has very *rough*, *dry skin* affecting the extensor surfaces of his arms. His trunk is less affected and his face is normal. He has *hyperpigmented palmar creases*. His eyes, mucous membranes and hair are normal. This boy has *ichthyosis*.

Notes

- Disorders of keratinization
- Two major forms are seen

Ichthyosis vulgaris

- Autosomal dominant
- Histology
  - absent epidermal granular layer
  - clinical
  - dry, rough skin, fine pale scales
  - extensor surfaces of arms most severely affected, face spared
  - improves in puberty
  - hyper-linear palms and plantar markings

Sex-linked ichthyosis vulgaris (ichthyosis nigricans)

- Sex-linked
- Only seen in males (female heterozygotes mildly affected)
- Presents at birth
- Aetiology
  - deficiency of steroid sulphatase
- Histology
  - increase in granular layer with an increased stratum corneum
- Clinical
  - large, greasy polygonal scales
  - scales mainly on the trunk and neck
  - palms and soles spared
  - corneal opacities occasionally seen

Defect may also affect placental steroid synthesis resulting in failure of onset of labour.

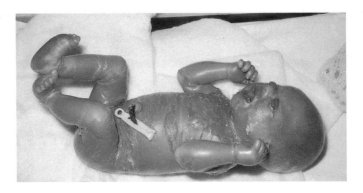

Fig. 21 'Collodian' newborn baby who subsequently developed typical skin changes of ichthyosis

Idiopathic thrombocytopaenic purpura

Examine this boy's skin

This young boy has *bruises* on both knees and has numerous *petechiae* over his body. There is no clinical evidence of anaemia. He has no active bleeding. I would like to make a full examination to exclude lymphadenopathy and hepatosplenomegaly. I would like to perform a FBC, blood film and coagulation screen. The most likely diagnosis in a well child with isolated thrombocytopenia is *idiopathic thrombocytopenia purpura*.

Notes

- Most common bleeding disorder of children
- Incidence = 1 : 25 000 children annually
- Platelet count < 100×10^9/l
- 80% of cases are preceded by viral illness (rubella, varicella, rubeola)
- Immune mediated – antibody vs platelet membrane glycoprotein
- Shortened platelet survival
- Spleen
  - site of sequestration of platelets
  - antibody production
- Incidence of intracranial haemorrhage – 0.1%
- Chronic ITP in 15% (platelet count decreased for 6 months)

Investigations

- FBC (platelets < 100×10^9/l)
- Coagulation (normal)
- Bleeding time ($\uparrow$)
- Immunoglobulins (platelet-associated IgG in 75%)
- Bone marrow ($\uparrow$ megakaryocytes)

Treatment

Acute ITP

- Nil needed usually
- Avoidance of situations likely to result in head injury
- Bone marrow sampling if diagnostic uncertainty
- Oral steroids – may cause more rapid rise in platelet count

- IVIG
  - active bleeding
  - failure to respond to steroids
  - cover for essential surgery
- Platelet transfusions only for life-threatening bleeding
- 90% remit spontaneously in 9–12 weeks

Chronic ITP

- All need bone marrow
- Need to exclude SLE and anti-phospholipid syndrome
- Splenectomy – only in those with significant symptoms 6 months from diagnosis. Mortality 1.5%

Incontinentia pigmenti (Bloch–Sulzberger disease)

Examine this young girl's skin

On inspection, this young girl has *cone-shaped teeth* and a *cataract* in her right eye. I note that she has had previous *cleft lip* surgery. She appears to have a *small head* and I would like to confirm this by measuring her OFC and plotting it on a growth chart. She has *bizarre hyperpigmented lesions* on her trunk that are brown and slate-grey in colour. Many of these lesions have a *whorled pattern*. My diagnosis is *incontinentia pigmenti*.

Notes

- X-linked dominant condition
- Usually lethal in males; 95% of cases are female
- Aetiology – 2 genes have been mapped
  - Xq28 – familial cases
  - Xp11 – sporadic cases

Three stages are seen:

1. Vesiculobullous stage
   - Present at birth or within 6 weeks of birth
   - Vesicles are scattered linearly on the lateral trunk and perimammary area
   - Vesicles may occur in utero
   - May last months
2. Verrucous stage
   - Begins within 2–6 weeks of birth
   - Seen in 60% of cases
   - Papules with a verrucous hyperkeratotic surface
3. Pigmentary stage
   - Begins in 12th–26th week of life
   - Seen in 100% of cases
   - Bizarre, macular hyperpigmented lesions that are brown, dirty brown and slate-grey
   - 'Whorled' pattern common
   - Patients may be born with hyperpigmented whorls (first 2 stages occur in utero)
   - Pigmentation fades after 2 years and by aged 20 most has disappeared
   - 14% develop areas of hypopigmentation

Defects

50% have other organ involvement:

- Dental defects – delayed dentition, pegged teeth, impactions
- Occular defects
  - seen in 30% of cases
  - strabismus, blindness, nystagmus, optic atrophy, uveitis, retinal pigmentation, blue sclera, retinal detachment
- Skeletal defects – skull deformities, dwarfism, spina bifida
- CNS defects – spastic paralysis, developmental delay, convulsions, slow motor development

Differential diagnosis

- Bullous impetigo
- Epidermolysis bullosa
- Candidiasis

Treatment

- Treatment of infections
- Dental treatment
- Family counselling

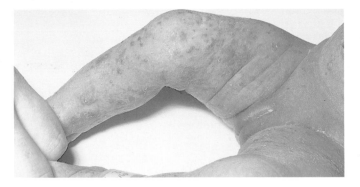

Fig. 22 Vesicular rash typical of incontinentia pigmenti in the early vesiculobulbous stage

Jaundice

Scenario I – What do you notice about this 2-month-old girl?

Jane is *jaundiced*! She is alert and looks well, although she does not have much subcutaneous fat (need to plot length, weight and occipito-frontal head circumference). She is not dysmorphic (Alagille and Zellweger syndromes), nor does she have features of congenital hypothyroidism (hoarse cry, coarse hair, cold, dry hands and feet). Abdominal system examination reveals a 5 cm *smooth hepatomegaly* below the right subcostal margin. There is no *splenomegaly or ascites*. Cardiovascular examination is important to exclude a cardiac defect seen with Alagille's syndrome (intra-hepatic biliary atresia and pulmonary stenosis – page 178).

Examination of the nappy demonstrates *white stools* and my primary concern is that this infant has extra-hepatic biliary atresia (EHBA). I would like to examine the urine (dark in EHBA because of bilirubin) and dipstick it for the presence of bilirubin and urobilinogen.

Notes

In infancy, the most likely diagnoses for obstructive jaundice with or without hepatomegaly and/or splenomegaly are:

- Cystic fibrosis
- EHBA
- Alagille's syndrome
- α1-antitrypsin deficiency
- Parenteral nutrition cholestasis

In the neonatal period, particularly in unwell babies, other diagnoses include:

- Neonatal hepatitis syndrome – CMV, Toxoplasmosis, Herpes
- Galactosaemia
- Congenital hypothyroidism
- Urinary tract infection

(It is very unlikely that you will see any of these in the exam.)

Guthrie card screening should exclude congenital hypothyroidism (and cystic fibrosis in regions measuring immunoreactive trypsin – Leeds, Trent, Norfolk, Wales).

Investigations, regardless of likely causation include urinalysis (bilirubin – EHBA; reducing substances – galactosaemia; nitrites, blood and organisms – UTI), split bilirubin (conjugated > 15–20% of total in obstructive jaundice) liver function testing (particularly ↑ ALT in EHBA), full blood count (WCC ↑ with infection), clotting studies (vitamin K deficiency), thyroid function tests, α1-anti-trypsin assay and phenotype, TORCH screen and galactose-1-phosphate uridyl transferase assay.

If EHBA is suspected, the infant needs a DISIDA scan ± a liver biopsy. Other possible investigations include a sweat test, metabolic screen (Zellweger's syndrome – see page 150), abdominal ultrasound (choledochal cyst).

Scenario II – What do you notice about this 10-year-old?

Janet (white) is *jaundiced*! She is also *Cushingoid*! (see page 78). There are stigmata of *chronic liver disease* present on her hands (palmar erythema, leuconychia, spider naevi) but no clubbing. Abdominal examination reveals a *non-tender splenomegaly* of 4 cm below the left subcostal margin. There is *no hepatomegaly* (because Janet has cirrhosis, but can be present, especially in disease with a less insidious onset, and may be tender), but there is *shifting dullness* suggesting ascites. There are no *surgical scars*. Although I can find no other evidence of autoimmune disease (vitiligo, erythema nodosum, thyroid or adrenal disease), the most likely diagnosis is autoimmune *chronic active hepatitis*.

Notes

- Patients with chronic active hepatitis may present with an acute hepatitis, chronic liver disease or fulminant hepatic failure
- In the majority of cases no cause is found and an autoimmune pathogenesis is presumed
- 50% present before the age of 20 years
- Cushingoid appearances can be as a result of chronic steroid administration or from Cushing's syndrome
- Other autoimmune diseases include arthritis, vasculitis, thyroiditis and nephritis.

Differential diagnosis

- Infective hepatitis – A, B, C, CMV, infectious mononucleosis
- α_1-anti-trypsin deficiency
- Sclerosing cholangitis – seen with inflammatory bowel disease
- Wilson's disease – see page 216
- Hereditary spherocytosis – see page 118

Investigations

These are similar to those for investigation of jaundice in a younger child. However, extra tests include – viral hepatitis serology, serum immunoglobulins ($\uparrow$ IgG), auto-antibodies (antinuclear, anti-smooth muscle, anti-mitochondrial, anti-liver/kidney microsomal, anti-thyroid antibodies and rheumatoid factor), direct Coombs' test. Liver biopsy.

Treatment

- High-dose oral steroids ± other immunosuppressive agents (principally azathioprine)
- Some patients do not respond to treatment and up to 70% relapse when treatment is weaned
- Transplantation may be necessary but recurrent disease can occur in the new liver

Juvenile chronic arthritis

Examine this girl's hands

She demonstrates symmetrical swelling of the wrists, metocarpophalangeal (MCP) joints and to a lesser extent, the proximal interphalangeal joints. There is *ulnar deviation* at the wrists and MCP joints. The overlying *skin is thin and shiny*, warm to the touch but not reddened. There is some *restriction of active movement* of the fingers, wrists and hands by the patient because of *pain* and *stiffness*. I will not attempt passive movements of these affected joints. Looking for other joint involvement, she has *swelling* and *deformity* of both knees, again without overlying skin colour changes. There is no rash present and she does not look systemically unwell (therefore not Still's disease). She is not overtly Cushingoid, but she has a full face and her skin is generally thin (chronic corticosteroid treatment). I would like to undertake an ophthalmic examination (cataracts, slit lamp examination required for detecting iridocyclitis [type I pauciarticular JCA]). I would also look for lymphadenopathy and splenomegaly. This girl has polyarticular *juvenile chronic arthritis*. Dipsticking the urine may reveal glucose (corticosteroids) or proteinuria (gold, penicillamine).

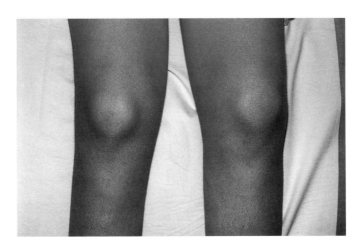

Figs 23–25 Juvenile chronic arthritis

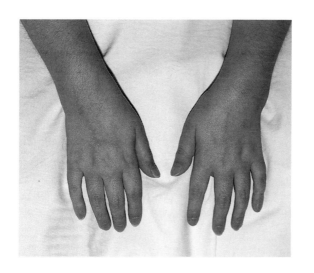

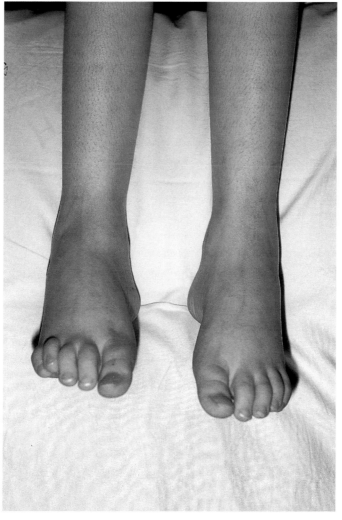

Notes

- Juvenile chronic arthritis encompasses a group of diseases with *chronic synovial inflammation* as the common theme.
- Causation is unknown

Still's disease – 20% of cases

- 1 male : 1 female
- Present with high swinging pyrexias, malaise, maculopapular rash and lymphadenopathy/hepatosplenomegaly
- The arthritis may not occur for several months after presentation
- Up to 60% will have pleuritis/pericarditis at presentation
- Rheumatoid factor and antinuclear antibody (ANA) negative

Polyarticular disease – 30%

- 1 male : 5 females
- Five or more joints are involved
- Can be divided into rheumatoid factor-positive and -negative disease. Those that are positive tend to have a more destructive course
- Iridocyclitis is rare

Pauciarticular disease – 50%

- Type I – 80% girls; positive ANA; a strong association with iridocyclitis
- Type II – 90% boys; association with HLA B27; iridocyclitis does not occur

Investigations

- Hb – low at presentation in Still's disease and in any chronic disease
- WCC and platelets – high at presentation in Still's disease
- ESR ↑ during active disease
- Rheumatoid factor, ANA
- HLA typing
- Immunoglobulins, complement
- X-rays

Differential diagnosis

- Leukaemia
- Neuroblastoma
- Systemic lupus erythematosis
- Lyme disease and other infections
- Dermatomyositis

Treatment

- Rest only in the acute phase
- Analgesia
- Anti-inflammatories
- 1st line – NSAIDs
- 2nd line – gold/penicillamine/hydroxychloroquine
- 3rd line – corticosteroids/azathioprine/methotrexate
- Splints/physiotherapy/occupational therapy
- Amyloid formation is rare but should warrant checking the urine for protein
- Annual ophthalmological examination should be undertaken in all children with JCA

Kawasaki disease

What do you think about this boy?

This miserable 3-year-old boy on general examination has bilateral non-purulent *conjunctival congestion, swollen, red and cracked lips* and a fine *polymorphous rash*. Further examination reveals tender cervical *lymphadenopathy* but none elsewhere and no splenomegaly. He has oedematous extremities with *erythematous* palms but no *desquamation* (a late sign of Kawasaki disease, but often the time when the diagnosis is thought of!). I would like to look into this child's mouth for the presence of mucosal erythema and 'strawberry' tongue. I would like also to measure his temperature and examine his cardiovascular system (tachycardia, gallop rhythm) including blood pressure. He fits the diagnostic criteria for *Kawasaki disease*.

Notes

- Acute febrile muco-cutaneous lymph node syndrome
- Incidence = 3–4 : 100 000 children < 5 years of age in the UK
- 1.5–2 males : 1 female; 75–85% of cases < 5 years of age
- Recurrent disease is described. Siblings of an index case are at higher risk than the general population
- A large number of organisms have been implicated, none are proven
- Vasculitis of the small and medium-sized arteries
- The commonest cause of acquired heart disease in children in the UK
- Mortality risk ~1% (treated), 20% (untreated)

Features

- Fever – unremitting, lasting longer than 5 days
- Bilateral conjunctival injection
- Oral changes – swollen, red or cracked lips, 'strawberry' tongue, mucosal erythema
- Peripheral extremity changes – erythema, oedema and desquamation
- Rash – polymorphous
- Cervical lymphadenopathy

A diagnosis is based on fever plus 4 of the other 5 features above.

- Miscellaneous – arthropathy, aseptic meningitis, mild obstructive jaundice, gallbladder hydrops

Investigations

- ESR ↑, platelets ↑, WCC ↑, CRP ↑
- ECG at diagnosis (prolongation of the PR interval, low voltages, ischaemic changes)
- ECG should be undertaken within 2 weeks from the start of the illness, 6 weeks later and at 6 months

Treatment

- Intravenous immunoglobulins – 2 g/kg over 8–12 hours
- High-dose aspirin – 30–100 mg/kg/day for 14 days or until the fever resolves, then 3–5 mg/kg/day, continued until cardiological assessment at 6–8 weeks

Differential diagnosis

- Staphylococcal scalded skin syndrome
- Toxic shock syndrome
- Leptospirosis
- Rickettsial infections

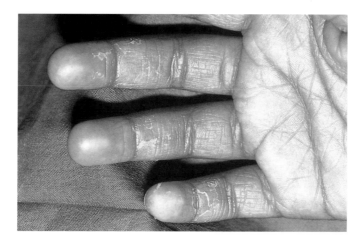

Fig. 26 Desquamation of the hands, seen after the first week of onset of the illness

Lobar pneumonia

Carry out a respiratory system examination

This 3-year-old girl is *dyspnoeic* at rest with a respiratory rate of 45 breaths per minute and a *cough*. She is not cyanosed, oxygen saturation is 94% in air (if attached to a monitor), but she does have mild *tracheal tug, sub-costal and inter-costal recession*. There is decreased chest wall movement on the right side of her chest and auscultation reveals coarse *crepitations* on this same side with *bronchial breathing* above. Attempts at percussion suggest *dullness* overlying this area. She does not demonstrate signs of chronicity such as clubbing or an abnormally shaped chest. Findings are consistent with a right-sided *lobar pneumonia*. She is too young to attempt eliciting whispering pectoriloquy. I would like to look at her temperature chart for evidence of a pyrexial illness.

Notes

- Most commonly occurs as a secondary bacterial infection following a viral respiratory illness unless there are underlying medical problems
- Look for stigmata of cystic fibrosis, immunodeficiency (e.g. eczema) or susceptibility for aspiration (nasogastric tube in situ)
- Can be associated with pleural effusion development (see page 166)

Differential diagnosis

- Bacterial – *Pneumococcus, Streptococcus, Staphylococcus, Klebsiella, Haemophilus*
- Viral – respiratory syncytial virus, Influenza, Coxsackie, adenovirus, CMV
- Others – Pneumocystis, Mycoplasma★, Chlamydia, Ureaplasma
- Inhalation of a foreign body with collapse/consolidation (may have mediastinal shift towards the affected side)
- Aspiration pneumonia
- Löffler's syndrome – eosinophilic pneumonia secondary to helminthic infection

★consider looking in the ears for bullous myringitis

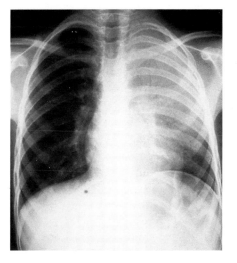

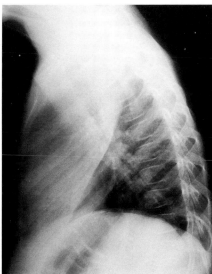

Figs. 27 & 28 A-P and lateral X-rays of complete left upper lobe consolidation

Lymphadenopathy

Examine the neck of this 3-year-old

On general inspection there are no obvious swellings, skin change or deformities of the neck. He has full range of passive movements without discomfort. On palpation (from behind) I can feel one discrete, non-tethered, non-tender lymph node, approximately 1 cm in diameter in the anterior cervical triangle. He looks systemically well, is not jaundiced (infectious mononucleosis) and has good nutritional status. There is no evidence of *lymphadenopathy* elsewhere (axillae, inguinal region) and no hepatosplenomegaly (80% of leukaemics have palpable splenomegaly at presentation). Looking in his mouth, he has large, non-inflamed tonsils (but no gum hypertrophy of acute leukaemia). Provided there is nothing else in the history to suggest otherwise (e.g. weight loss, lethargy, night sweats, contact with tuberculosis), I think this is *reactive lymphadenopathy* and does not warrant investigation, but simple follow-up.

Notes

- If there is parental concern, ask them (or the GP) to monitor the size of the lymph node over time
- If in doubt a full blood count is very reassuring (to exclude leukaemia particularly)
- Other investigations may be indicated if any of the conditions below are suspected

Causes

- Infectious – glandular fever, Streptococcal throat infections, TB, atypical mycobactria
- Collagen disorders – JCA (page 134), SLE, Sjögren's syndrome
- Malignancies – ALL, lymphoma
- Miscellaneous – Kawasaki disease (page 138), sarcoid, drugs

Macrocephaly

What do you want to examine with this boy?

This baby boy appears to have a disproportionately large head and plotting his height, weight and occipito-frontal head circumference (largest of three measurements) confirms *macrocephaly*. He shows no evidence of dysmorphology. Examination of the spine again reveals no abnormalities (looking particularly for spina bifida).

Notes

The rate of growth of head circumference is more important than a one-off measurement. Up to 1 cm/week head growth is expected in well premature babies, but only 0.4 cm/week in term babies. Catch-up head growth occurs after chronic illness.

Differential diagnosis

Is it normal, brain, bone, marrow or fluid?
- Normal variation
- Familial macrocephaly – autosomal dominant, measure parental head circumference and plot
- Bone disorders – rickets, osteogenesis imperfecta, achondroplasia (see page 36)
- Cerebral neoplasms – glioma, ependymoma

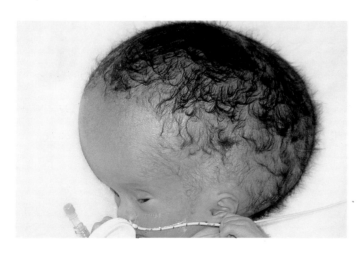

Fig. 29   Post-haemorrhagic hydrocephalus secondary to prematurity

- Megalencephaly – tuberous sclerosis (see page 219), neurofibro-matosis (see page 155), mucopolysaccharidoses (see page 123), Tay–Sachs disease, leucodystrophies, Soto's syndrome
- Space-occupying lesions – haematoma, sub-dural and epidural effusion, hydranencephaly, holoprosencephaly
- Bone marrow expansion – thalassaemia
- Hydrocephalus – communicating or non-communicating. Splaying of the sutures, bulging fontanelle, distended scalp veins and 'sun-setting' eyes

Investigation

- Measurement of parental and sibling OFC
- FBC and Hb electrophoresis – marrow causes
- Liver function tests, calcium profile – bone causes
- Cranial ultrasound scan ± CT scan ± MRI scan – normal, brain and fluid causes
- Skull and skeletal survey if bone disorders considered likely
- Enzyme assays on cultured skin fibroblasts – mucopolysaccharidoses, Tay–Sachs disease

---

Comment on this boy's facial appearance

This boy has no obvious dysmorphic features. He does, however, have a large protruding tongue. He has no suggestion of cardiorespiratory distress at rest in air (obstruction of the upper airway). He has *macroglossia*.

Notes

The differential diagnoses for macroglossia include:

1. Physiological
2. Down's syndrome – see page 88 (normal-sized tongue in small mouth)
3. Mucopolysaccharidoses, e.g. Hurler's syndrome. See page 123
4. Hypothyroidism
5. Pompe's disease
   - Glycogen storage disease Type II – Autosomal recessive
   - Chromosome 17
   - Affected enzyme – α,1,4-glucosidase (acid maltase)
   - Can present in neonatal period, infancy or adulthood
   - Features
     - affects all organs
     - generalised muscle weakness
     - failure to thrive
     - hepatomegaly
     - hypertrophic obstructive cardiomyopathy
     - short PR interval
     - huge QRS complex
     - heart failure. Death usually by age 1 due to heart failure.
   - Diagnosis
     - enzymatic study of lymphocytes, muscle or skin fibroblasts
     - vacuolated lymphocytes in blood film
   - Treatment
     - bone marrow and cardiac transplant – unsuccessful
     - high protein diet may improve muscle weakness
     - enzyme replacement in future may be a possible
6. Beckwith–Wiedemann syndrome
   - Aetiology – mostly sporadic, 15% are familial
   - Genetics – imprinted genes from chromosome 11
   - Features
     - macrosomia

- gigantism
- macroglossia
- facial naevus flammeus in centre of forehead
- prominent eyes
- renal dysplasia
- diaphragmatic eventration
- cryptorchidism
- exomphalos
- linear fissures on external ear lobe
- indentations on posterior rim of helix
- pancreatic hyperplasia resulting in hyperinsulinaemic hypogly-caemia in 50%
- mild to moderate mental retardation rare – severe in poorly treated hypoglycaemia
- Associated with hemihypertrophy – 20%
- Tumours seen in 5% – hepatoblastoma, Wilm's tumour, adrenal carcinoma, gonadoblastoma

7. Lymphangioma
8. Haemangioma
9. Rhabdomyoma
10. Cystic hygroma

Marfan's syndrome

Examine this lad's hands and proceed as you deem appropriate

This adolescent boy appears tall for his age (needs to be plotted accurately on the appropriate centile chart) with *disproportionate limb length*. He has *arachnodactyly* of his fingers and toes with a positive wrist sign (ability to encircle their own wrist with 5th finger and thumb of the opposite hand) and *Steinberg sign* (thumb adduction across the palm of the same hand). He has a high, arched palate and hyper-extensible joints. All these features are suggestive of a connective tissue disorder. Auscultation of the praecordium reveals a pan-systolic murmur heard loudest at the apex with radiation to the axilla and a mid-diastolic murmur suggestive of *mitral regurgitation*. He wears spectacles because of myopia and demonstrates *iridodenesis*. This child has probable *Marfan's syndrome*.

Notes

- Incidence = 1 : 10 000; 1 male : 1 female
- Autosomal dominant, 25% of cases are new mutations
- Chromosome 15 – deletions of the fibrillin-1 gene
- Reduced tissue elasticity because of abnormal fibrillin production affecting skin, tendons, muscle, blood vessels, pleura, periosteum, cartilage and ciliary zonules
- Marfan's syndrome is a clinical diagnosis because each family carries a unique mutation

Skeletal system

- Arm span is greater than height (> 90%)
- Arachnodactyly (> 90%)
- High, arched palate (> 90%)
- Tall stature (> 80%)
- Pectus deformity – carinatum or excavatum (80%)
- Pes planus (80%)
- Scoliosis (50%)

Eyes

- Iridodenesis/dislocated lens
- Myopia
- Blue sclera

Cardiovascular

- Aortic root dilatation (80%)

- Mitral valve prolapse – mid-systolic click +/− late systolic murmur
- Mitral valve incompetence – left parasternal heave, 3rd heart sound, pan-systolic murmur

Miscellaneous

- Striae
- Herniae – inguinal
- Spontaneous pneumothorax
- Poor muscle development with hypotonia
- Decreased subcutaneous fat

Follow-up

- Annual echocardiography, slit lamp examination of eyes, orthopaedic review
- Avoidance of strenuous exercise advisable

Prognosis

- Death due to cardiovascular complications, usually before age 50
- β-blockers may improve survival
- Elective surgery for aortic root dilatation

Differential diagnosis

- Homocystinuria (autosomal recessive)
  - developmental delay
  - downwards lens dislocation
  - osteoporosis
  - malar flush
- Klinefelter's syndrome see p 207
  - small testes
  - no cardiac/ophthalmological complications

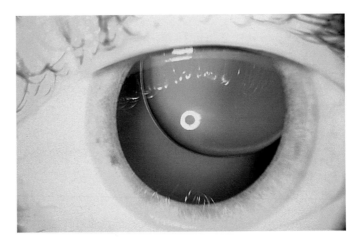

Fig. 30 Lens dislocation (upwards) in Marfan's syndrome

- Ehlers–Danlos syndrome see p 96
- McCune–Albright syndrome
- Multiple endocrine neoplasia type 3 – marfanoid habitus, thickened lips, ectropion, lip and tongue nodules (ganglioneuromas)

Microcephaly

Examine this baby's head

This boy appears to have a small head with backward sloping of the forehead. He has no other dysmorphic features. I would like to confirm that his head is small by measuring occipitofrontal circumference (OFC) and plotting it on an appropriate growth chart. I would like to perform a full neurological and developmental examination. The diagnosis is *microcephaly*.

Notes

Definition: OFC > 3 standard deviations below the mean for age and sex.

Aetiology

1. Normal variation – need to measure weight and height, and plot on suitable growth chart
2. Familial – autosomal recessive, dominant. Need to measure parental OFC and plot
3. Genetic disorders:
   - Prenatal chromosomal – Trisomy 21, 13, 18
   - Partial deletion – e.g. cri du chat
4. Malformation – Lissenencephaly, schizencephaly
5. Syndromes
   - Cornelia de Lange syndrome (see page 70)
   - Rubenstein–Taybi syndrome (see page 187)
   - Prader–Willi syndrome (see page 171)
   - Seckel's syndrome
   - Zellweger's syndrome
     - cerebrohepatorenal syndrome
     - autosomal recessive
     - incidence = 1 : 100 000
     - absence of peroxisomes resulting in accumulation of very long-chain fatty acids
     - high foreheads, microcephaly, flat orbital ridges, wide opened fontanelle and sutures, hepatomegaly, renal cortical cysts (97%), hypotonia, abnormal liver function tests
     - stippled calcification of patella and acetabulum on X-ray
     - Diagnosis – elevated VLCFA in serum; liver biopsy
6. Intrauterine infections – TORCH infections

7. Toxins
   - Maternal pelvic radiation
   - Maternal alcohol ingestion
   - Maternal PKU
8. Metabolic
   - Phenylketonuria
     - autosomal recessive
     - incidence = 1 : 10 000
     - absence of phenylalanine hydroxylase
     - developmental delay, fair hair, eczema, blue eyes, microcephaly, fits, cerebral palsy. Autistic behaviour. Mousy smelling urine
     - Guthrie card measures phenylalanine
     - Treatment – Low phenylalanine diet
   - Hypoglycaemia
   - Maple syrup urine disease
     - autosomal recessive
     - incidence = 1 : 200 000
     - deficiency of branched chain ketoacid dehydrogenase
     - hypoglycaemia, ketoacidosis, seizures, caramel smell
     - raised blood and urine leucine, isoleucine and valine levels
9. Perinatal hypoxia – neonatal hypoxic-ischaemic injury
10. Craniosynostosis
    - Apert's syndrome (see page 73)
    - Crouzon's syndrome (see page 73)
11. Perinatal infection
    - Meningitis (group B Streptococcus)
    - Viral encephalitis (coxsackie B)

Investigation for a child with microcephaly

- Full history, including family history
- Full examination, especially cataracts, hepatosplenomegaly, skin rashes
- Skull imaging
- Maternal phenylalanine level
- Chromosome studies
- Blood
  - toxoplasma antibody titres
  - CMV IgM titres
  - rubella IgG and IgM titres
- Urine – CMV
- Throat swab – viral culture

Myotonic dystrophy (Steinert's disease)

Examine this boy's face

This boy has *bilateral ptosis*. He has bilateral *facial weakness* and is unable to screw his eyes up completely and bury his eyebrows. He has an inverted *V-shaped upper lip* and wasted facial, temporalis, masseter and sternomastoid muscles. He speaks with a *nasal voice*. I would like to examine him for evidence of *myotonia* (slow relaxation after contraction – unable to open hand quickly after making a fist) and *percussion myotonia* (depressions induced in his thenar muscle by percussion are very slow to fill). I would like to examine his testicles for evidence of gonadal atrophy. My diagnosis is *myotonic dystrophy*.

Notes

- Autosomal dominant inheritance with anticipation (see genetics below)
- Chromosome 19
- Incidence = 1 : 8000
- Neonatal and juvenile forms seen

Other features

- Hypotonia
- Cataracts
- Frontal baldness
- Gonadal atrophy (85%)
- Thyroid dysfunction
- Cardiac dysrhythmia
- ↓ IgG
- Diabetes mellitus (due to end organ resistance to insulin)
- Developmental delay
- ↓ life expectancy

Investigations

- EMG – spontaneous myotonic discharges with gradual decrement (With sound amplification it resembles a departing motor bike)
- Serum CK: normal (or slightly ↑)
- Muscle biopsy – Type 1 muscle fibre atrophy

Neonatal form (congenital)

- Infants born to mothers with myotonic dystrophy
- Majority dead by end of 1st year (respiratory failure)
- Features
  - facial weakness
  - poor swallowing/feeding
  - ptosis
  - tented upper lip (fish-shaped mouth)
  - absent Moro reflex
  - poor respiration
  - congenital contractures
  - talipes of feet
  - history of polyhydramnios (poor fetal swallowing)
  - poor fetal movements
  - prolonged labour
- Diagnosis – made by demonstrating myotonia in mother (shake hands with mother)
- Investigations – as above

Genetics

- Instability in a CTG repeat sequence present in the 3′ untranslated region of a protein kinase (DMPK)
- Normal unaffected person – CTG sequence consists of 30–35 repeats
- Affected person – CTG sequence consists of 50–2000 repeats
- More severe forms have the largest number of repeats

Anticipation

The disease occurs at an earlier age and with increasing severity in the offspring than the parents (due to expansion of the CTG triplet repeat). Also seen in Huntington's disease, Fragile X syndrome.

Nephrotic syndrome

Look at this boy's face – what do you want to do?

This young boy has prominent peri-orbital oedema and appears *Cushingoid*. Further examination reveals *dependent pitting oedema* of his lower limbs, scrotal and prepuce oedema. He also demonstrates *abdominal striae, ascites* and *tender smooth hepatomegaly*. Examination of his respiratory system is unremarkable. The presence of *xanthomas* around his eyes suggests *hypercholesterolaemia*.

The findings are consistent with a diagnosis of *nephrotic syndrome*. Urinalysis to demonstrate *proteinuria* would be useful.

Notes Hypoalbuminaemia

- Hypoproteinaemia (< 25 g/l), proteinuria and oedema
- Investigation – U&Es, LFTs, ANF, ds-DNA antibodies, hepatitis serology, complement, urine microscopy and electrophoresis
- Renal biopsy in children over 10 years? Minimal change nephropathy less likely if < 1 year old or older than 10 years.
- Treatment with high-dose steroids, penicillin, no added sodium diet and fluid restriction if grossly oedematous. The vast majority are steroid-sensitive. Renal biopsy if steroid-resistant at 28 days of treatment.
- Complications – arterial and venous thrombosis, bacterial infections (particularly *Streptococcus*). Subcapsular cataract formation with prolonged steroid use

Differential diagnosis

- Minimal change nephropathy 85%
- Focal segmental glomerulonephritis (GN) 10%
- Mesangiocapillary GN in 5%
- In older children and adults think of HSP, SLE, amyloid and drugs

Neurofibromatosis

Look at this young lady's arms

On first inspection this adolescent girl has several subcutaneous swellings with poorly defined margins on her limbs. The overlying skin is hyperpigmented and hairy. Further examination of the skin reveals *axillary freckling* and at least 10 hyperpigmented areas distributed about the body. The presence of these *plexiform neurofibroma*, axillary freckling and *café au lait* spots makes the diagnosis of *neurofibromatosis type 1* (NF1) very likely. Confirmatory evidence would include the presence of: *lisch nodules* (which may require slit lamp examination to confirm their presence); short stature; *macrocephaly*; and the development of dermal neurofibromas in later childhood and adulthood. A search for stigmata of neurofibromatosis in family members is essential. To complete my examination I would like to measure her blood pressure (*phaeochromocytoma, renal artery stenosis*).

Notes

- Incidence = 1 : 2500–3000; 2 males : 1 female
- Autosomal dominant inheritance, 50% represent new mutations
- Chromosome 17
- NF1 gene encodes for the protein neurofibromin that is involved in the regulation of ras in the cell that controls cell development and division. In effect, the NF1 gene acts as a tumour suppressor gene.

Major features – very variable

- Six or more *café au lait* spots (> 5 mm in diameter before puberty, > 15 mm post-puberty)
- Two or more neurofibromas or one plexiform neurofibroma
- Axillary and/or inguinal freckling
- Optic glioma
- Two or more Lisch nodules (iris hamartomas)
- First-degree relative with NF1

Other features

- Macrocephaly – 50%
- Short stature – 30%
- Learning difficulties – 30%
- Developmental delay – 8%

- Miscellaneous
  - phaeochromocytoma
  - renal artery stenosis
  - aqueductal stenosis
  - scoliosis
  - CNS tumours
  - glaucoma
  - coloboma
  - hemihypertrophy

Follow-up

- Annual review of symptoms and blood pressure check
- Specialist combined clinics (paediatrician, neurologist, dermatologist, neurosurgeon, psychologist, ophthalmologist) are increasingly common

Differential diagnosis

- Proteus syndrome ('elephant man')
- Congenital generalised fibromatosis
- McCune–Albright syndrome
- LEOPARD syndrome – (see page 180)
- Schimke osseus dysplasia

> N.B. *Café au lait* spots are also seen in Fanconi's anaemia, Russell–Silver syndrome (see page 193), tuberous sclerosis (see page 202), Chediak–Higashi syndrome (autosomal recessive, oculocutaneous albinism, killer cell deficiency, recurrent infections, malignancies), Bloom syndrome (autosomal recessive, telangiectasia of the face, short stature, malignancies, chromosomal fragility) and ataxia telangectasia.

Neurofibromatosis type 2

- This is a separate disease entity
- Chromosome 22
- Incidence = $1 : 50\ 000$
- Unilateral or bilateral acoustic neuromas (more correctly vestibular Schwannomas) in adulthood plus meningiomas and spinal tumours
- Lisch nodules, developmental delay, bone disease and phaeochromocytomas are not seen in NF2.

Segmental or mosaic NF1 describes patients with one or more features of NF1, particularly *café au lait* spots, limited to isolated body dermatomes.

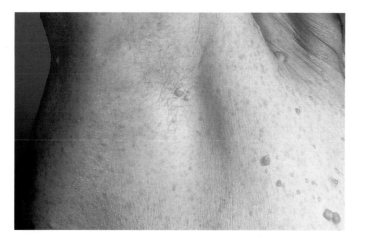

Fig. 31 Typical skin changes in NF1

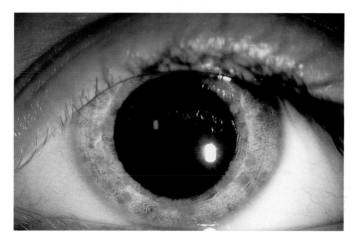

Fig. 32 Lisch nodules

Optic atrophy

Examine this girls' eyes

On retinal examination, this girl has bilateral, very pale but distinct optic discs. There are no changes suggestive of papilloedema or hypertensive retinopathy. *Visual acuity* is markedly reduced, more prominently centrally than peripherally. I would like to go on and perform a full neurological examination to see if an underlying causation can be found for her *optic atrophy*.

Notes

- Primary or secondary
- Primary causes – Leber's hereditary optic atrophy
- Secondary causes – congenital, degenerative, inflammatory, vascular or neoplastic

Specific causes

- DIDMOAD – diabetes insipidus, diabetes mellitus, optic atrophy and deafness. Test the hearing and look for injection sites
- Friedreich's ataxia – spinocerebellar degeneration presenting with clumsiness, scoliosis, pes cavus, intention tremor, nystagmus, incoordination, loss of reflexes, explosive dysarthric speech, extensor plantar responses and loss of position and vibration sense
- Laurence–Moon–Biedl syndrome (see retinitis pigmentosa, page 183)
- Behr's autosomal recessive optic atrophy – hypertonia, developmental delay and ataxia
- Tay–Sachs disease
- Zellweger's disease

Osteogenesis imperfecta

Comment on this boy's appearance

This young boy has a plaster cast on his right arm. He appears short and I would confirm this by plotting him on a centile chart. He has a marked *scoliosis*. His *sclerae are blue*. I note that his father has blue sclerae and bilateral hearing aids. The most likely diagnosis is *osteogenesis imperfecta*.

Notes

- Incidence = 1 : 20 000 births
- Pathology – abnormality in one of the three α chains that form the triple helix of type I collagen resulting in fragile, matrix-depleted bones
- Blue sclerae due to choroidal pigment showing through thinned sclera

Type 1

- Autosomal dominant (10% sporadic)
- Mild to moderate disease
- Blue sclerae after 6 months
- Hypotonia
- Hypermobile joints
- Otosclerosis (deafness in 40% by 40)
- Herniae
- Small stature due to bony deformity
- Wormian bones (> 10 measuring 6 × 4 mm needed to be significant)
- Aortic/mitral valve prolapse
- Scoliosis
- Bowing of limbs
- Abnormal dentition (dentinogenesis imperfecta) in 50% – Type 1B (Type 1A – normal dentition)

Type 2

- Autosomal dominant (some recessive)
- Lethal disease
- Stillborn or neonatal death
- All have numerous fractures at birth
- Short, bowed limbs
- Narrowed deformed chest
- Blue sclerae

Type 3

- Autosomal dominant
- Moderate to severe disease
- Blue sclerae
- Bowed limbs
- Wormian bones
- Death aged 20–30

Type 4

- Autosomal dominant
- Moderate severe disease
- Normal sclerae, normal teeth, normal hearing

Differential diagnosis of blue sclerae

- Ehlers–Danlos syndrome, see page 96
- Incontinentia pigmenti, see page 129
- Marfan's syndrome, see page 147
- Russell–Silver syndrome, see page 193
- Pseudoxanthoma elasticum

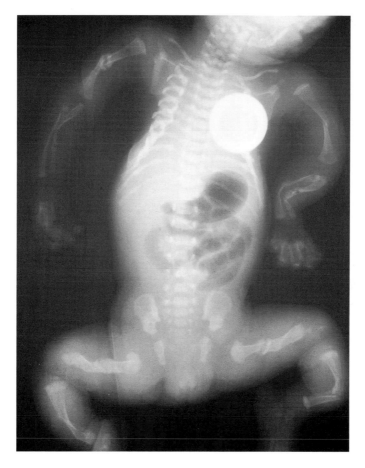

Fig. 33 X-ray demonstrating multiple bone fractures in a lethal form of osteogenesis imperfecta

Papilloedema

Look in this girl's eyes

This 6-year-old girl has markedly dilated pupils, presumably after instillation of mydriatic agents. Retinal examination demonstrates bilateral *blurring* and *heaping* up of the optic nerve disc margins, reddening of the discs (*hyperaemia*) and *loss of pulsation* of the retinal veins (!). There are no flame-shaped haemorrhages (but these can be seen with *papilloedema*). Visual acuity (Snellen chart) and colour vision (Ishihara charts) are normal (unlike with optic neuritis). This child has *optic nerve swelling* and requires investigation to exclude intracranial pathology. I would like to go on and look at the other cranial nerves (particularly for a lateral rectus palsy – abducens nerve) and perform a full CNS examination. I would also measure the *systemic blood pressure* using the appropriately sized cuff.

Notes

- Papilloedema is defined as optic nerve swelling secondary to raised intracranial pressure
- Intracranial pathology is suspected until proven otherwise

Differential diagnosis

- ↑ ICP – tumour, thrombosis, hydrocephalus, infection
- Orbital – tumour, abscess, uveitis
- Benign intracranial hypertension – 50% have an unknown causation, the rest secondary to drugs, infection, endocrinopathies, haematological problems

It is important to differentiate papilloedema from the retinal changes of hypertension. These include increased retinal artery tortuosity and reflectiveness (silver wiring), A–V nipping, flame-shaped haemorrhages and soft exudates.

N.B. Papilloedema does not occur in the first 12–18 months of life until the cranial sutures are fused.

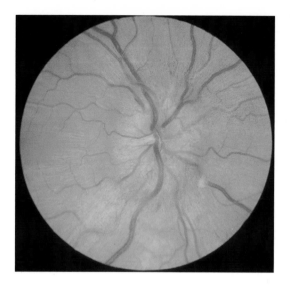

Fig. 34 Papilloedema

Petechial rash

Examine this boy's skin

This boy has numerous petechiae and purpura covering much of his skin.

Notes

- Most common causes in childhood are trauma, Henoch–Schönlein purpura, ITP and leukaemia
- Petechiae < 1 mm in diameter; purpura 1–10 mm in diameter; ecchymosis > 10 mm in diameter

Differential diagnosis of petechial/purpuric rash

1. Abnormalities of vascular endothelium
   - Trauma
   - Henoch–Schönlein purpura (see page 112)
   - Infection (meningococcus)
   - Connective tissue disease (SLE)
   - Scurvy
   - Ehlers–Danlos syndrome (see page 96)
2. Platelet disorders

Decreased platelet production
   - Megakaryocyte failure (post viral)
   - Bone marrow infiltration
     - leukaemia
     - neuroblastoma

Increased destruction of platelets
   - Immune – idiopathic thrombocytopaenic purpura (see page 127)
   - Consumption – disseminated intravascular coagulation
   - Haemolytic uraemic syndrome
   - Giant haemangiomas, e.g. Kasabach–Merritt syndrome
   - Hypersplenism
     - haematological (spherocytosis)
     - malignancy (lymphoma)
     - infection (infectious mononucleosis)
     - metabolic (Gauchers)
   - Infection – CMV, rubella

Abnormal platelet function
   - Drugs (NSAIDS)

- Uraemia
- Von Willebrand's disease
- Bernard–Soulier syndrome

3. Coagulopathy
   - Inherited – Haemophilia A (Factor VIII), Haemophilia B (Factor IX)
   - Acquired – DIC, liver disease

4. Congenital disorders

Wiskott–Aldrich syndrome
- X-linked recessive
- Incidence = 1 : 4 million males
- Features
  - thrombocytopenia
  - eczema
  - immune deficiency (recurrent otitis media)
- Immunoglobulins – $\uparrow$ IgA, $\uparrow$ IgE, $\downarrow$ IgM
- Increased autoimmune disease – haemolytic anaemia, vasculitis, arthritis
- Increased malignancy – non-Hodgkin's lymphoma
- Treatment
  - active bleeding – irradiated platelets
  - HLA-matched bone marrow transplant from matched sibling donor

Bernard–Soulier syndrome
- Autosomal recessive
- Moderate bleeding tendency resulting in recurrent bruising and purpura
- Giant platelets on blood film. Increased bleeding time
- Inherited deficiency of platelet membrane glycoprotein 1b leading to absent aggregation with ristocetin
- Frequent platelet transfusions needed but may develop antibodies against glycoprotein 1b of transfused platelets

Kasabach–Merritt syndrome
- Large cavernous haemangioma (skin or abdominal viscera) associated with thrombocytopenia and evidence of intravascular coagulation
- Most common sites are limbs and limb girdles
- Consumption of platelets and coagulation factors in haemangiomas

Thrombocytopenia with absent radii syndrome (TAR syndrome)
- Severe thrombocytopenia associated with aplasia of the radii and thumbs
- Isolated failure of platelet production
- Occasionally seen: cardiac and renal anomalies
- Usually presents in neonatal period – 35% mortality in 1st year
- Transfused platelets have normal survival

Pleural effusion

Examine this boy's chest

This 10-year-old boy is clubbed and has an abnormally shaped chest with increased A–P diameter and Harrison's sulci. His resting respiratory rate is 30 breaths per minute. He has moderate intercostal recession and decreased chest wall movement on the left side. Percussion note is dull at the left base but resonant elsewhere. Auscultation reveals decreased air entry over this area of *dullness* with *bronchial breathing* above it. There is no evidence of tracheal deviation or cyanosis. He has a dressing over his ribs in the mid-axillary line (pleural tap). A history of cough, fever and malaise together with the mentioned signs make the diagnosis of *pleural effusion* secondary to underlying pneumonia likely. The presence of clubbing suggests *co-existent pathology* such as cystic fibrosis.

Notes

Pleural effusion warrants an attempt at diagnostic tap in all cases. This will differentiate between an exudate and transudate but more importantly may be diagnostic if due to an infective cause.

Differential diagnosis

- Causes besides pneumonia are likely to have other symptoms and signs
- Left-sided heart failure
- Nephrotic syndrome – generalised oedema, proteinuria, hypoproteinaemia
- Tuberculosis – night sweats, weight loss
- Malignancy – rare
- Hypothyroidism – rare

Poland anomaly

Examine this boy's upper body

On inspection this boy has an abnormally shaped *flattened chest wall* on the left and ipsilateral fusion of the fingers of his left hand (*syndactyly*). The diagnosis is *Poland anomaly*.

Notes

- Aetiology – sporadic
- Embryology – vascular interruption in 6th week of development
- Incidence
  - 1 : 20 000
  - 4 males : 1 female
  - 75% of defects on the right

Features

- Aplasia of pectoralis major muscle (sternocostal portion) and pectoralis minor
- Hypoplasia of nipple and areola occasionally seen
- Varying degrees of ipsilateral syndactyly/brachydactyly also found
- Ipsilateral hypoplasia of kidney and hemivertebrae occasionally seen
- Normal life expectancy
- Reconstructive surgery

Other conditions with hand abnormalities

1. Thrombocytopenia-absent radii (TAR) syndrome – see page 165
2. Fanconi's anaemia
   - Autosomal recessive
   - Absent/hypoplasia of thumbs, radius
   - Aplastic anaemia
   - Short stature
   - Microcephaly
   - Developmental delay
   - Bilateral hearing loss
   - Café au lait spots (ragged outline)
   - Renal anomalies (absent, hypoplasia, horseshoe)
   - Cryptorchidism
   - Ptosis
   - ↑HbF

- ↑red cell MCV
- ↑ chromosomal breaks
- Treatment – bone marrow transplant

3. Blackfan–Diamond syndrome
   - Red cell aplasia
   - Absent/hypoplastic thumbs
4. Holt–Oram syndrome – see page 120

Polycystic kidney disease

Examine this girl's abdomen

This girl appears *short* and she is *pale*. She has a *peritoneal dialysis catheter in situ* and bilateral flank masses. On palpation she has bilateral renal enlargement and 6 cm hepatomegaly. The diagnosis is *polycystic kidney disease*. I would like to check her blood pressure.

Notes

Infantile polycystic kidney disease
- Incidence = 1 : 40 000 live births
- Aetiology
  - autosomal recessive
  - gene on chromosome 6
- Pathology
  - cysts occur in the cortex and medulla representing dilatation of the collecting ducts. The cysts are fusiform in shape and radially orientated so that the overall 'reniform' shape is preserved
  - the liver shows evidence of fibrosis from a young age
- Clinical
  - bilateral renal enlargement (kidneys may fill abdominal cavity)
  - cysts may be large enough at birth to obstruct labour
  - oligohydramnios may be present in utero
  - gross haematuria, hypertension, failure to thrive, renal failure are seen
  - severe cases present with Potter's syndrome with pulmonary hypoplasia
  - most common presentation is respiratory failure. Renal function may be impaired at birth
- Renal USS – bright echogenic microcysts
- Renal IVP – opacification of the collecting ducts and presence of 'radial streaks'
- Problems – cirrhosis, portal hypertension, and cholestasis
- Treatment
  - supportive
  - treatment of chronic renal failure and hypertension
  - transplantation

Adult polycystic kidney disease
- Incidence = 1 : 200–1000
- Aetiology

- autosomal dominant
- two genes
  i. PKD 1 – chromosome 16 (short arm); 90% of cases; gene closely linked to α haemoglobin gene
  ii. PKD 2 – chromosome 4 (long arm)
- Pathology
  - cysts occur in any part of the nephron
  - irregular distribution of cysts throughout the cortex and medulla
  - kidneys asymmetrical in size
- Clinical
  - microscopic haematuria, hypertension, flank pain, proteinuria, renal failure. Children may present with unilateral/bilateral flank masses
  - uncommon to have symptoms in childhood (symptoms rare < 20 years)
  - can present in neonates (very severe)
  - 10% have cysts by 10 years old
  - 95% have cysts by 19 years old
  - end-stage renal disease aged 60–70
- Associated – cerebral artery aneurysms

N.B. To distinguish between infantile and adult PCKD, it may be worthwhile obtaining a renal ultrasound of the child's parents. Adult PCKD is autosomal dominant and so parents may have asymptomatic signs.

> ## What do you think is wrong with this boy?
>
> This 9-year-old boy is markedly *overweight* and appears short for his age. To differentiate between simple obesity and the *Prader–Willi syndrome* I would expect to find *developmental delay*, *micropenis* and *cryptorchidism* in boys, together with a history of poor feeding and *generalised hypotonia in infancy*. Children with PWS often start walking late because of the severe hypotonia that gradually resolves over the first year of life. Plotting this child's height on the appropriate centile chart will demonstrate short stature that is in contrast to simple obesity in which pre-pubertal children are often tall for their age. Retinal examination to exclude retinitis pigmentosa and the Laurence–Moon–Biedl syndrome is essential.

Notes

- Sporadic
- 55–70% have interstitial deletion of 15q 11–13 from the paternally inherited chromosome 15 (see Angelman's syndrome, page 38)
- 5% have duplications or translocations
- 45% normal karyotype, some of whom have maternal uniparental disomy, i.e. 2 normal chromosome 15s passed inherited from their mother
- Obesity classically develops after the 1st year of life secondary to insatiable appetite, inactivity and low resting energy requirements

Features

- Characteristic facies – anti-mongoloid slant to the eyes, 'carp-like' mouth
- Scoliosis – common in adolescence
- Insulin resistance and diabetes mellitus
- 'Pickwickian syndrome' and cor pulmonale
- Delayed secondary sexual development
- Small hands and feet
- Hypertension

Differential diagnosis

1. Obesity
   - Tall for age (pre-pubertal)
   - Early secondary sexual development

2. Laurence–Moon–Biedl syndrome
   - Short stature
   - Hypogonadism
   - Obesity after the 1st year of life and developmental delay as in PWS, **but** retinitis pigmentosa, polydactyly and diabetes insipidus
3. Smith–Magenis syndrome (17p–)
   - Phenotypically similar to PWS but children demonstrate self-destructive behaviour

Prune belly syndrome

Examine this boy's abdomen

On abdominal system examination, this boy has obvious deficiency of *abdominal wall musculature*. There is no palpable bladder, organomegaly or ascites. He has *bilateral undescended testes*, but has what appears to be a patent penile urethra. To confirm the triad of findings described in Prune belly syndrome I would undertake imaging of this boy's renal tract. I would also like to measure his *blood pressure*, assess renal function and culture his urine to exclude a urinary tract infection.

Notes

- Abdominal wall musculature deficiency
- Undescended testes
- Renal tract muscle deficiency

Features

- Urethral atresia
- Patent urachus
- Intestinal malrotation
- Asymmetrical lower limbs and reduction deformities

Aetiology

- Temporary urethral obstruction in the 1st trimester of pregnancy causing dilatation of the renal tract with abnormal function

Treatment

- Surgical correction of the undescended testes
- Prophylactic antibiotics to prevent renal tract infection
- Surgical intervention of the renal tract abnormalities rarely indicated

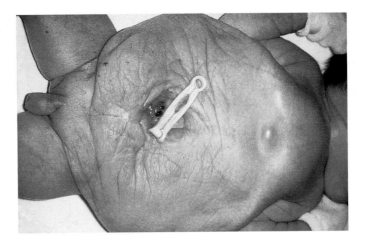

Fig. 35 Prune Belly syndrome

Psoriasis

> ## What do you think about this girl's skin?
>
> This 15-year-old girl has a widespread *erythematous papular rash* affecting all areas including the face and scalp but not the soles, palms or mucous membranes. The lesions are confluent in the intertriginous areas and are *centripetal* in distribution. Scratching the surface of the lesions reveals an underlying silver plaque. The lesions are *itchy* and there is evidence of scratching. The adolescent's hair is normal and there is no pitting of her nails. I would like to examine all her joints for evidence of *arthropathy*. She has *guttate psoriasis*.

Notes

- One-third of psoriasis sufferers present before adulthood
- In children, the first presentation is commonly as guttate psoriasis following a streptococcal throat infection and less commonly following measles
- Common plaque psoriasis may follow on from the guttate form or be the initial presentation. Occasionally napkin dermatitis is due to psoriasis and may require skin biopsy to differentiate it from chronic fungal or inflammatory causes. Other forms include psoriatic erythroderma, flexural (inverse) and palmoplantar psoriasis
- Common plaque psoriasis has a strikingly symmetrical distribution
- The *Koebner phenomenon* can be seen in 40–50% (also seen in lichen planus, lichen sclerosus, molluscum contagiosum)
- Psoriasis has a multifactorial inheritance pattern. Guttate and common plaque psoriasis and psoriatic erthyroderma are more common in people with HLA-B13 and HLA-B17
- Nail involvement is common (reported frequency in childhood from 14–79%). Nail pitting, onycholysis, sub-ungual hyperkeratosis, thickening and crumbling are all seen

Differential diagnosis

1. Infant psoriasis
   - Nappy area – fungal dermatitis
   - Scalp – seborrhoeic dermatitis, tinea capitis, Langerhan's cell (class 1) histiocytosis (formerly called Letterer–Siwe histiocytosis)
2. Acute guttate psoriasis
   - Drug eruptions, pityriasis rosea (look for a herald patch)

Treatment

- Avoidance of skin injury (Koebner response)
- Psychosocial support (lifelong condition, no cure)
- Topical therapies
  - anthralin (Lasser's paste)
  - coal tar preparations
  - corticosteroids
- Systemic therapies (not recommended in children)
  - methotrexate
  - retinoids
- Photochemotherapy – psoralen and longwave ultra-violet-A therapy (PUVA)

Ptosis

Examine this boy's eyes

On inspection, this boy has bilateral drooping of both eyelids. I would like to continue by examining his visual fields, visual acuity, eye movements and pupillary reflexes. To finish I would like to perform fundoscopy. The diagnosis is *bilateral ptosis*.

Notes

Ptosis can be unilateral, bilateral, congenital or acquired.

Congenital ptosis
- Most common anomaly of eyelids
- Unilateral or bilateral
- Aetiology
  - autosomal dominant familial ptosis
  - fetal alcohol syndrome
  - myotonic dystrophy
  - Aarskog's syndrome
  - Moebius syndrome
  - Noonan's syndrome – see page 222
  - Rubenstein–Taybi syndrome – see page 187
  - Smith–Lemli–Opitz syndrome
  - incomplete development of levator muscle
  - congenital defect of 3rd cranial nerve
  - 3rd cranial nerve trauma at birth
  - Marcus Gunn jaw winking – ptosis improves on opening mouth. Aetiology: 5th cranial nerve supplies levator muscle

Acquired ptosis
- Aetiology
  - physiological
  - myasthenia gravis – see page 104
  - myotonic dystrophy – see page 152
  - trauma
  - inflammation
  - botulism
  - brain stem tumour
  - dermatomyositis
  - Kearn–Sayre syndrome (mitochondrial myopathy)

Pulmonary stenosis

Examine the cardiovascular system

This child is pink in air with no evidence of cardiovascular distress and no finger clubbing. Heart rate is 80 beats per minute, of normal volume and character. The apex beat is not displaced but a *right para-sternal heave* is noted consistent with *right ventricular hypertrophy*. Palpation over the pulmonary region (2nd intercostal space, left sternal edge) demonstrates a *systolic thrill*, grade 4/6. Auscultation reveals the 1st heart sound, with splitting of the 2nd (quiet pulmonary component) due to delayed closure of the pulmonary valve. There is an *ejection systolic murmur* heard loudest over the pulmonary region with radiation throughout the praecordium. To complete my examination I would look for evidence of cardiac failure (hepatomegaly, peripheral and pulmonary oedema) and measure the blood pressure. This child has *pulmonary stenosis*.

Notes

Pulmonary stenosis can occur in association with a right to left shunt across an atrial or ventricular septal defects. Clinical features are dependent upon the degree of stenosis and size of the left to right shunt, but the child may be cyanosed with finger clubbing.

Causes
- Congenital valvular pulmonary stenosis
- Noonan's syndrome
- William's syndrome (see page 230)
- Alagille's syndrome (see page 179)
- LEOPARD syndrome (see page 180)
- Tetralogy of Fallot (see page 101)
- Congenital rubella syndrome (pulmonary arterial branch stenosis)

Investigations

- CXR – cardiomegaly, prominent right ventricle (± right atrium), decreased pulmonary vascular markings if significant right to left shunt)
- ECG – right ventricular hypertrophy and prominent P waves (right atrial hypertrophy)
- Echocardiography
- Angiography – a systolic gradient of over 50–60 mmHg between the

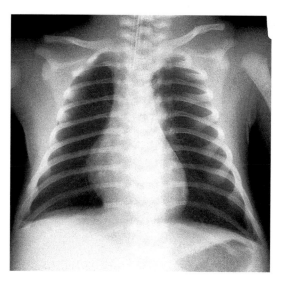

Fig. 36 X-ray showing prominent right ventricle and oligamic lung fields

right ventricle and pulmonary artery at rest with a normal cardiac output requires valvotomy or surgery

Differential diagnoses

1. Noonan's syndrome
   - Normal karyotype
   - Short stature
   - Webbed neck
   - Pectus deformities
   - Cubitum valgus
   - Hypertelorism
   - Antimongoloid slant
   - Micrognathia
   - 25% with developmental delay
   - Cryptorchidism in boys
2. Alagille's syndrome
   - Autosomal dominant
   - Chromosome 20
   - Intrahepatic cholestasis
   - Peripheral pulmonary stenosis (or tetralogy of Fallot)
   - Soft dysmorphic features and vertebral arch defects (hemi- or butterfly vertebrae)
   - A child with Alagille's syndrome may have signs of drug induced immunosuppression (cushingoid with steroids, lanugo hair with cyclosporin) and a transverse abdominal wall surgical scar from liver transplantation (25% of cases)

3. LEOPARD syndrome
   - **L**entigines
   - **E**CG abnormalities
   - **O**cular hypertelorism
   - **P**ulmonary stenosis
   - **A**bnormal genitalia (cryptorchidism)
   - **R**etardation of growth
   - **D**eafness (sensorineural)
4. Congenital rubella syndrome
   - Microcephaly
   - Developmental delay
   - Hearing loss
   - Cataracts

Renal transplant

Examine this young boy's abdomen

On inspection this young boy is small and I would like to confirm this by plotting him on an appropriate growth chart. He has a round flushed face and is *hirsute* (cyclosporin side effect). He has a small linear scar over his left wrist (*haemodialysis fistula operation*). On inspection of his abdomen he has a gastrostomy and a *peritoneal dialysis catheter*. There is an obvious scar in the right iliac fossa overlying a small mass. On palpation of his abdomen there is no hepatosplenomegaly and I cannot feel his kidneys. He has a mass in his right iliac fossa, which is firm, smooth, fixed, and non-tender. This boy has had a *renal transplant*. He is *Cushingoid* probably as a result of steroids. I would like to check his blood pressure.

Notes

Rental transplantation is the optimal treatment for end-stage renal disease. Underlying pathology in children with renal transplant:

- Obstructive nephropathy
- Renal aplasia/dysplasia
- Focal and segmental glomerulosclerosis
- Reflux nephropathy

Immunosuppression

Many drugs are used including:

Corticosteroids
- Side-effects – see page 79

Azathioprine
- Side-effects
  - bone marrow suppression
  - hypersensitivity

Cyclosporin
- Side-effects
  - nephrotoxicity
  - hypertrichosis
  - gingival hypertrophy

Tacrolimus
- Used as primary immunosuppression and in rejection
- Side-effects
  - cardiomyopathy
  - leucocytosis
  - leucopenia

OKT3
- Used in rejection
- Monitor CD3 + T-cells

Outcome
- 3-year graft survival
  - living donor kidney – 80%
  - cadaveric kidney – 65%

Retinitis pigmentosa

Carry out fundoscopy

Examination of this 14-year-old boy reveals black pigmentation of the retina primarily involving the peripheries. The macula and its immediate surroundings are spared but the optic disc appears pale. Further ophthalmological examination demonstrates a loss of peripheral vision. I note that his mother has significant visual impairment (white stick, guide dog!) and suspect that she too may have *retinitis pigmentosa*.

Notes

- Autosomal recessive, dominant or sex-linked inheritance
- Presents initially with night blindness, progressing to tunnel vision and eventual blindness
- No treatment available
- Electroretinography is indicated if RP is suspected.

Secondary pigmentation of the retina occurs in a number of conditions mimicking primary retinitis pigmentosa. These include:

1. Laurence–Moon–Biedl syndrome – very similar clinical picture to Prader–Willi syndrome
   - Autosomal recessive
   - Obesity
   - Polydactyly
   - Hypogonadism
   - Developmental delay and growth delay (secondary to growth hormone deficiency)
   - Association with diabetes insipidus
2. Refsum's disease
   - Phytanic acid hydroxylase defect resulting in phytanic acid deposition in peripheral nerves (polyneuropathy)
   - Retina (pigmentation)
   - Cerebellum (ataxia)
   - Heart (cardiomyopathy)
   - VIIIth cranial nerve (deafness)
   - Autosomal recessive inheritance
   - Treatment with a phytanic acid restricted diet
3. Abetalipoproteinaemia
   - Fat malabsorption due to an inability to form LDL, VLDL and chylomicrons from apoprotein B deficiency

- Results in fat-soluble vitamin deficiencies (vitamin K – bleeding tendencies; vitamin E – retinal pigmentation, cerebellar ataxia; vitamin D – rickets; vitamin A – xerophthalmia); acanthocytosis of the red blood cells
- Children present with failure to thrive, diarrhoea/steatorrhoea and ataxia
- Look particularly for an intention tremor, loss of position and vibration sense (posterior column involvement)
- Treatment with high doses of fat-soluble vitamins and a low-fat diet

4. Mucopolysaccharidoses – see page 123

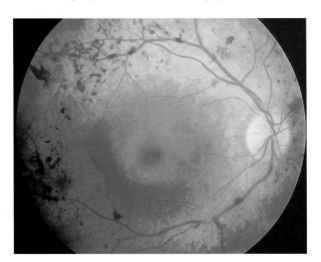

Fig. 37 Retinitis pigmentosa

Notes

- Sporadic occurrence
- Affects females only
- Incidence = 1 : 15 000
- Aetiology unknown
- Responsible for 25–33% of severely developmentally delayed girls
- Normal development to 1 year of age followed by a global regression of skills including receptive and expressive language, social interactions and fine motor skills
- Deceleration of head growth
- Loss of purposeful hand skills at age 1–4 and development of stereotypic hand movements including hand wringing, hand-washing (invisible soap), hand-tapping, hand-to-mouth (hand-wetting) movements. Hands kept at chest or chin level
- Short stature with small hands and feet
- Scoliosis seen in most girls by age 11
- Other orthopaedic complications seen include: equinovarus deformity, fractures due to osteopenia
- Breathing pattern abnormalities: hyperventilation and breath holding/apneoic episodes
- Teeth-grinding, facial grimacing seen in 90% of girls
- Wide-based, stiff-legged gait if girl can walk
- Fits seen in 75% of affected girls
- High pain threshold – secondary to elevated β-endorphin levels in CSF
- Cold clammy peripheries – secondary to increased sympathetic tone
- No characteristic laboratory abnormality
- CT/MRI shows cerebral atrophy
- EEG may be normal or show frequent sharp waves localised to central/Sylvian regions

Differential diagnosis

1. Angelman's syndrome – see page 38

2. Joubert's syndrome
   - Autosomal recessive
   - Episodic hyperpnoea (panting dyspnoea)
   - Jerky eye movements
   - Ataxia
   - Mental retardation
   - Retinal dysplasia
   - Hemifacial spasms
   - CT – absence of cerebellar vermis, umbrella-shaped 4th ventricle
3. Infantile autism
   - Affects 2–10 : 10 000
   - 3 males : 1 female
   - Characterised by language abnormalities, social abnormalities and prominent repetitive or ritualistic behaviours

Rubenstein–Taybi syndrome

Comment on this boy's appearance

This boy is *short* and has *microcephaly*. I would like to confirm this by plotting him on an appropriate growth chart. He has *ante-mongoloid slant of the palpebral fissures* and his eyes are set wide apart (*hypertelorism*). He has *posteriorly rotated ears, a beak-shaped nose* and a *prominent forehead*. His *thumbs and halluces are very broad*. He is *developmentally delayed*. To complete my examination and confirm the diagnosis I would like to examine his cardiovascular system for any evidence of *congenital heart disease*, which has an increased incidence in this condition. I would also like to examine his genitalia for *undescended testes*. The findings are consistent with a diagnosis of *Rubenstein–Taybi syndrome*.

Notes

- Microdeletion
- Chromosome 16
- IQ is usually less than 50

Features

- Strabismus
- Large anterior fontanelle
- Ptosis
- Hirsuitism
- Kyphoscoliosis
- Clinodactyly
- Radially deviated thumbs
- Heart defects (VSD, ASD, PDA)
- Renal anomalies

X-rays

- Delay of ossification
- Occasional abnormalities of pelvis/thorax/vertebral column

Scoliosis

Examine this girl's back

This girl appears well and has no dysmorphic features. Examination of her back in the standing position demonstrates that she has a marked mid-thoracic *scoliosis* convex to the right. On bending forward the scoliosis is exaggerated and she has a marked *hump* of her right posterior ribs. I would next like to examine her spine with her sitting down to eliminate unequal leg length followed by a full neurological examination including gait. I would finally like to make a full examination of the cardiorespiratory system for complications of scoliosis.

Notes

Scoliosis — lateral curvature of the spine with rotation. Can occur in thoracic or lumbar spine.

- Curvature described by direction of convexity
- Kyphosis: posterior curvature of spine (normal in thoracic area)
- Lordosis: anterior curvature of spine (normal in lumbar area)

Aetiology of scoliosis

Postural
- 2° to leg length inequality, muscle weakness
- Disappears on forward flexion and on sitting

Structural

Idiopathic — 80%
- Infantile
  - 0- to 3-year-olds; males > females
  - thoracic most common, convex to left in > 80%
- Juvenile
  - 4- to 10-year-olds; males = females
- Adolescent
  - > 10-year-olds; 7 females : 1 male
  - mid-thoracic most common, convex to right in 90%

Congenital — 7%
- Hemivertebrae, wedge vertebrae

Neuromuscular — 10%
- Neurofibromatosis — see page 155

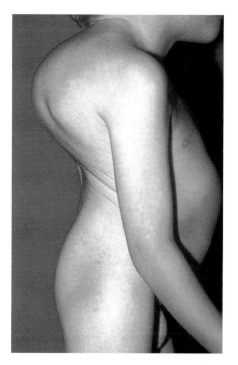

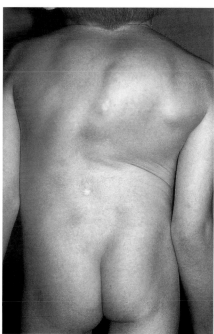

Figs 38 & 39   Scoliosis

- Cerebral palsy
- Muscular dystrophy – see page 91
- Poliomyolitis
- Myelomeningocele
- Friedrich's ataxia – see page 40
- Spinal muscular atrophy

Miscellaneous – 3%
- Marfan's syndrome – see page 147
- Trauma
- Osteogenesis imperfecta – see page 159

Scrotal swelling

Comment on this infant's perineum

This 2-month-old boy has non-tender, right-sided *scrotal swelling*. The swelling is soft, *fluctuant* and *transilluminates* (due to the thinness of the bowel wall). It is not possible to feel above the swelling within the scrotal sac (unlike a hydrocele), but 'milking' of the mass caudally and laterally towards the inguinal canal results in its disappearance. Increasing intra-abdominal pressure (by tickling the baby and making them laugh; alternatively make the baby cry, but not recommended for the exam! Rarely will a baby cough spontaneously for you!) results in an increased size and firmness of the mass. Apart from the swelling I note that the infant requires supplemental oxygen via nasal cannulae and has a dolicocephalic-shaped head consistent with prematurity.

In summary, this boy has a right-sided reducible *inguinal hernia*.

Notes

- 12 males : 1 female
- Two-thirds right-sided, ~5–7% bilateral
- Predisposing factors
  - cryptorchidism
  - congenital dislocation of the hip – 3× more likely
  - prematurity (13% of infants < 2000 g, 19% of infants < 1500 g, 30% of infants < 1000 g)
  - ascites
  - chronic lung disease, e.g. bronchopulmonary dysplasia, cystic fibrosis
  - mucopolysaccharidoses – Hunter's syndrome, Hurler's syndrome
  - connective tissue diseases – Ehlers–Danlos syndrome see page 96
  - renal dysplasia, bladder exstrophy

Inguinal herniation occurs because of persistence of the processus vaginalis that normally obliterates in the third trimester of pregnancy after testicular descent into the scrotum.

Treatment

- Herniotomy ± exploration of the contra-lateral side
- Because of the risk of incarceration early surgical intervention should be undertaken

- For a hydrocele, the majority disappear spontaneously and should therefore not be treated surgically under one year of age

Differential diagnosis

- Non-tender – hydrocele
- Tender
  - torsion of the testes
  - epididymo-orchitis – mumps, chlamydia, gonorrhoea

N.B. In females with inguinal/labial swelling, consider the diagnosis of testicular feminisation syndrome and the presence of testicular tissue.

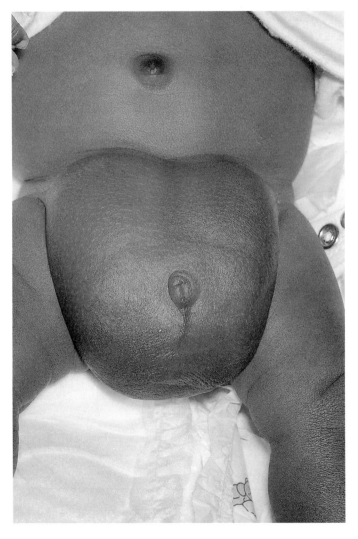

Fig. 40   Bilateral reducible inguinal hernias in a premature infant

Short stature

> ## Comment on this girl's appearance
>
> This young girl appears very *short*. I would like to measure her accurately and plot her on a centile chart. The diagnosis is *short stature*.

Notes

Aetiology
1. Constitutional
   - Delayed growth
   - Delayed bone age
   - Normal height attained
2. Familial
   - Parents are short
   - Bone age consistent with actual age
   - Normal height velocity
3. Malnutrition
4. Endocrine
   - Hypothyroidism
   - Hypopituitarism
   - Cushing's syndrome (including iatrogenic)
   - Diabetes mellitus (poorly controlled)
   - Growth hormone deficiency
5. Metabolic
   - Rickets
   - Hypercalcaemia
   - Storage disorders (mucopolysaccharidoses, mucolipidoses)
6. Skeletal dysplasia
   - Achondroplasia (see page 36)
   - Osteogenesis imperfecta (see page 159)
   - Albright's hereditary ostrodystrophy
7. Syndromes
   - Turner's syndrome (see page 221)
   - Noonan's syndrome (see page 222)
   - Prader–Willi syndrome (see page 171),
   - Laurence–Moon–Biedl syndrome (see page 183)
   - Russell Silver Dwarf
     - aetiology – sporadic
     - small triangular face
     - small chin
     - frontal bossing

- café au lait spots
- clinodactyly
- hypoglycaemia in infancy
- normal IQ
- Aarskog's syndrome
  - hypertelorism
  - cryptorchidism
  - shawl scrotum
8. Chronic conditions
   - Cardiovascular
     - congenital heart disease
   - Respiratory
     - cystic fibrosis (see page 80)
   - Gastroenterology
     - malabsorption
     - coeliac disease (see page 62)
     - Crohn's disease/UC (see page 76)
   - Haematology
     - thalassaemia (see page 209)
     - sickle cell disease (see page 195)
   - Nephrology
     - chronic uraemia
     - renal tubular acidosis

Sickle cell disease

> **Examine this boy's abdomen**
>
> This *Afro-Caribbean* boy is *pale*. He appears to be *short* but I would confirm this by plotting him on an appropriate growth chart. His nail beds are pale and he has a painful swollen finger on his right hand. On palpation of his abdomen he has a mass in the left upper quadrant that moves with respiration, has a notch on its medial border and is dull to percussion. I cannot get above the mass. (*Splenomegaly* only present below 5 years of age – 'auto-splenectomy' occurs.) My diagnosis is *sickle cell disease* with *dactylitis*.

Notes

- Autosomal recessive
- Disorder of haemoglobin synthesis due to a single base mutation of adenine to thymine that results in a single amino acid substitution (valine for glutamine) at the 6th codon of the β-globin chain
- In the UK – 15% of Afro-Caribbeans carry the gene

Homozygote

Sickle cell anaemia (HbSS) – HbA (0%), HbS (90%), HbA$_2$ (2–3%), HbF (5–15%). HbSS presents after 6 months of age (when HbF levels $\downarrow$)

Heterozygote

Sickle cell trait (HbAS) – HbA (55–60%), HbS (40–45%), HbA$_2$ (2–3%)

Pathology

- De-oxygenated HbS molecules $\rightarrow$ distorting of RBC (sickling) resulting in: $\uparrow$ blood viscosity, capillary obstruction, $\downarrow$ RBC survival to 20 days (normal – 120 days)
- Exacerbating sickling – dehydration, infection, hypoxia and acidosis
- HbAS – asymptomatic unless hypoxic

Clinical – HbSS

Anaemia

- Chronic haemolytic anaemia (Hb 5–9 g/dl), $\uparrow$ reticulocyte count (5–15%)
- Film: nucleated RBC, target cells, sickle cells, Howell–Jolly bodies (hyposplenism)

Infection

- Sickling of RBC in spleen → splenic dysfunction → inability to filter microorganisms → infection. Recurrent sickling results in splenic infarction and eventually → autosplenectomy (therefore spleen not palpable after 5 years old)
- Infection especially with encapsulated organisms: *S. pneumoniae, H. influenzae, Salmonella*

Splenic crisis

- Hyperacute fall in Hb due to blood pooling in the spleen

Aplastic crisis

- Infection with human parvovirus B19 → transient red cell aplasia

Painful crisis

- Due to vaso-occlusion
- Occurs in hands (dactylitis), penis (priapism), avascular necrosis of femoral head, muscle, bone marrow, intestines
- Leg ulcers

Acute chest syndrome

- Cyanosis
- Fever
- Chest pain
- Dyspnoea
- Thrombocytopenia

Gall bladder disease

- Cholecystitis
- Gallstones

Growth

- Reduced growth
- Delayed puberty

Renal

- Papillary necrosis
- Haematuria
- Nocturnal enuresis (loss of concentrating ability due to recurrent infarcts)

Eye

- Retinal detachment

Splenomegaly

Examine this boy's abdomen

On inspection, this boy has *tortuous dilated veins* radiating over the abdomen from the umbilicus and a full-looking abdomen. On palpation there is a mass in the left hypochondrium that extends down towards the right iliac fossa. The mass moves with respiration and I cannot get above it. It is dull to percussion and has a notch on its medial side. On percussion his abdomen is dull in both flanks, which becomes resonant on lying him on his side. The diagnosis is *splenomegaly* with *portal hypertension*.

Notes

Causes

1. Infection
   - Bacterial – septicaemia, TB, bacterial endocarditis, brucella
   - Viral – infective hepatitis, infectious mononucleosis, CMV
   - Protozoal – malaria, toxoplasmosis
2. Haematology
   - Severe Fe anaemia
   - Sickle cell anaemia
   - Spherocytosis
   - Thalassaemia
3. Infiltration
   - Malignancy – lymphoma, leukaemia, Histiocytosis X
   - Storage disorders
4. Portal hypertension – see below
5. Connective tissue disease
   - Still's disease
   - SLE

Portal hypertension

- Most common cause of splenomegaly
- Normal portal venous pressure: 5–10 mmHg, portal hypertension: > 10 mmHg

Aetiology

Pre-hepatic

- Portal vein obstruction – history of neonatal sepsis, umbilical vein catheter sepsis

Hepatic
- Cirrhosis
- Congenital hepatic fibrosis
- Cystic fibrosis

Post-hepatic
- Hepatic vein occlusion (Budd–Chiari syndrome)
- Raised vena caval pressure
  - congestive cardiac failure
  - constrictive pericarditis

Clinical features

- Ascites
- Splenomegaly
- Portal-systemic venous collaterals (oesophageal varices, caput medusae and haemorrhoids)

Squint

> ## I have been asked to examine this 1-year-old boy's eyes
>
> I can find no obvious abnormalities on initial inspection (e.g. dysmorphic features, broad epicanthic folds, manifest squint, coloboma, cataract, proptosis, ptosis). The boy is alert and fixes on my face. Testing for visual acuity demonstrates that he can see tiny objects (try rolling brightly coloured balls of progressively smaller size along the floor). Visual fields appear intact because his eyes turn to the finger puppet (or other such interesting object!) when introduced in all areas of vision. He follows the puppet in all areas. The reflection of a pen torch light from his cornea is symmetrical and he therefore does not have a manifest *squint*. Performing the cover–uncover test for a squint reveals a *latent convergent squint* of the left eye. I cannot report on his fundoscopy findings because he finds it hard to sit still and his pupils are not dilated (but I would dilate the eyes and look again for completion). I would complete my examination of the eyes with testing of the corneal reflex. He has a latent convergent *squint* of the left eye and formal visual acuity testing is required to exclude hypermetropia.

Notes

Be wary of the child with a false eye! Always test visual acuity first. In an older child get them to hold a book (so that you can see how far they hold it from their face as an indication of far- or near-sightedness) and get them to read. Whilst doing this, cover up each eye in turn to see if they continue reading!

Squint (strabismus) can be defined as existing when both visual axes do not intersect the point of visual attention. It can be classified into paralytic and non-paralytic. Non-paralytic squints are convergent, divergent or alternating. Paralytic squints are due to IIIrd, IVth or VIth nerve palsies. It is concomitant if the abnormal angle between the visual axes remains approximately constant in all directions of gaze, i.e. the non-paralytic squints.

IIIrd nerve palsy

The eye looks down and out, the pupil can be dilated, there is ptosis, absent pupillary reflexes and eye movements are very limited. Remember that the third cranial nerve originates in a series of mid-brain nuclei, passes through the cavernous sinus along its lateral wall to enter the orbit through the superior orbital fissure to supply the superior, medial and inferior recti, the inferior oblique and the levator palpebrae superioris muscles. It also carries pre-ganglionic parasympathetic fibres.

IVth nerve palsy

Result in diplopia on looking down and in (classically patients have problems walking downstairs). The trochlear nerve has a similar route to the IIIrd cranial nerve and supplies the superior oblique.

VIth nerve palsy

Produces a lateral rectus palsy. Arises from the pons, leaves the brain stem, passing over the petrous temporal bone, through the lateral aspect of the cavernous sinus to enter the orbit, again through the superior orbital fissure.

Visual acuity

Adult visual acuity (6/6) is not attained until 2 years of age. At birth it is 3/60, at 6 months 6/30 and at 18 months 6/9.

Squint can be dealt with in four ways

- Occlusion (wearing a patch over the good eye)
- Ocular exercises
- Surgical correction
- Wearing of prescription glasses

Swollen knee

> ## Examine this young boy's knee
>
> This boy has a *swollen right knee*. His knee is red, warm and tender to the touch. He is in pain through a full range of active and passive movements. He has a positive patellar tap and therefore a knee effusion. I would like to look at the child's temperature chart, examine his other knee for comparison and examine his gait. I would also like to make a full examination of the child's skin for a rash and also his nails.

Notes

Aetiology
1. Trauma
   - Most common cause of swollen joint.
   - History of trauma. (N.B. NAI)
2. Infection
   - Bacterial
     - febrile child
     - swollen joint
     - reluctance to weight bear
     - ↑ WCC, ↑ PV, ↑ ESR, ↑ CRP, blood cultures
     - joint ultrasound
     - joint X-ray
     - aspiration of joint
     - organisms: *Staphyloccus aureus*, coliforms, *Haemophilus influenzae*, *Salmonella*, TB
   - Post-viral
     - rubella
     - CMV
     - mumps
     - chicken pox
     - adenovirus (transient synovitis, reactive arthritis)
   - Rheumatic fever
     - Group A β-haemolytic streptococcus
     - arthritis (large joints)
     - carditis
     - rheumatic nodules
     - erythema marginatum
     - Sydenham's chorea (minor – ↑ ESR, fever, arthralgia, previous RF, prolonged PR on ECG)
   - Spirochaetal – Lyme disease – *Borrelia burgdorferi*

- Rickettsial – Rocky mountain Spotted Fever
3. Connective tissue disease
    - Henoch–Schönlein purpura – see page 112
    - Systemic lupus erythematosus
    - Juvenile chronic arthritis – see page 134
4. Inflammatory bowel disease
    - Ulcerative colitis – see page 76
    - Crohn's disease – see page 76
5. Malignancy
    - Leukaemia
6. Haematological
    - Haemophilia A, B
    - Sickle cell disease – see page 195
7. Psoriasis
    - Examine skin, scalp, nails
8. Dermatomyositis – see page 84

Syndactyly

Comment on this boy's appearance

This boy is short and obese and I would like to confirm this by plotting him on an appropriate growth chart. He has bilateral fusion of the fingers of both hands (*syndactyly*). Given the presence of syndactyly in a short, obese child, the diagnosis of *Laurence–Moon–Biedl syndrome* is likely and I would like to confirm this by examining his genitalia for hypogonadism and performing fundoscopy to look for *retinitis pigmentosa*.

Notes

Syndactyly
- Most common congenital anomaly of the hand
- Incidence = 1 : 2200
- May involve many degrees of fusion from simple webbing of the skin to full bony fusion

Syndromes with syndactyly
- Apert's syndrome – see page 73
- De Lange syndrome – see page 70
- Holt–Oram syndrome – see page 120
- Orofaciodigital syndrome
- Polysyndactyly
- Fetal hydantoin syndrome
- Fanconi's pancytopenia
- Trisomy 13
- Trisomy 18
- Trisomy 21 – see page 88
- Laurence–Moon–Biedl syndrome (see page 183)

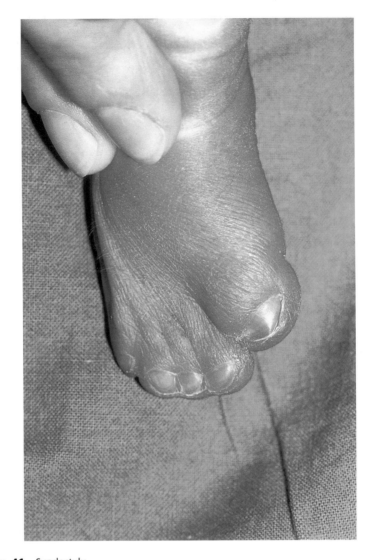

Fig. 41 Syndactyly

Talipes equinovarus

Examine this boy's foot

This boy has *fixed plantar flexion* of his foot, *inversion of the heel, hindfoot and forefoot* and *adduction of the forefoot*. The diagnosis is *talipes equinovarus*. I would like to make a full examination of his spine and hips.

Notes

- Incidence = 1 : 1000 live births
- 2 males : 1 female
- 50% of cases are bilateral

The shape of the foot is secondary to medial dislocation of the talonavicular joint

Aetiology

- Positional
  - secondary to in utero position
  - associated with oligohydramnios
- Congenital
  - 75% of cases
  - usually an isolated abnormality
  - isolated risk is 0.1%
  - if one parent has condition risk is 3–4%

Associated with

- Neuromuscular disorders
- Myelomeningocele
- Poliomyelitis
- Cerebral palsy
- Myelodysplasia
- Arthrogryposis multiplex congenita
- Congenital hip dysplasia

All children with talipes equinovarus must have a full examination with special attention to the spine.

Treatment

- Massage, manipulation to stretch the contracted tissues on the medial and posterior aspects of the foot, adhesive strapping
- Surgical release may be needed in some cases

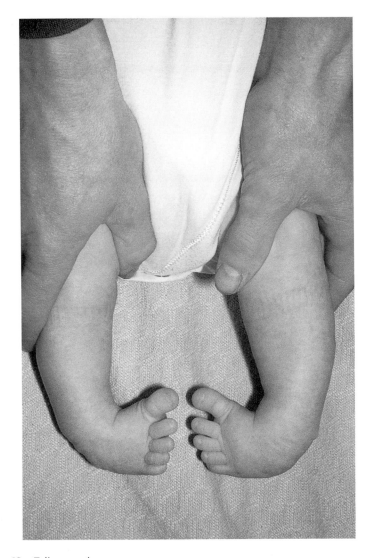

Fig. 42   Talipes equinovarus

What do you notice about this boy?

The most striking feature about this 14-year-old boy is his standing height. He appears to be well over 6 feet tall and of relatively slim build. I note that his mother is not particularly tall and it would be very useful to know his father's height. He appears to have *disproportionate tall stature* and to confirm I will measure his upper segment (US) to lower segment (LS) ratio (upper segment = height − lower segment; lower segment = symphysis pubis to the floor). A normal US:LS after the age of 8 should be no less than one.

There are no obvious signs of puberty, i.e. no facial hair, his voice is still unbroken, and (if allowed to demonstrate this, using a goniometer) testicular volume is around 2 ml with no pubertal enlargement of the penis. However, he does have pubic hair development. Talking with James, I suspect that developmentally he may be a little behind, with poor attention span and this certainly warrants further formal assessment.

The findings may simply represent constitutional delay of growth and development but because of his tall stature and the loss of consonance I am concerned about *Klinefelter's syndrome*.

Notes

- Incidence = 1 : 1000 male births
- Due to non-disjunction of an X chromosome, in two-thirds of cases from the mother
- Besides 47XXY, other variants can occur, e.g. 48XXXY, 49XXXXY
- ~1% of all people with developmental delay may have Klinefelter's syndrome or a variant
- Diagnosis is by chromosomal analysis
- Pubertal gynaecomastia is a common occurrence
- Tall stature results from delayed fusion of the long bone epiphyses (because of very low testosterone secretion). Growth hormone therefore continues to exert its effects on long bone growth
- Puberty is not delayed but testicular volume does not increase appropriately, nor does penile length. It is this loss of consonance that should make one undertake appropriate investigations

Differential diagnosis

- Constitutional delay of growth and development

- Gonadotrophin deficiency
- Marfan's syndrome – see page 147. Test quickly for hyper-extensibility and look for arachnodactyly
- Hyperthyroidism – see page 213. Measure the heart rate, feel the hands for increased temperature and sweating and look at the neck and eyes for positive signs
- Neurofibromatosis type 1 – see page 155
- McCune–Albright syndrome
- Soto's syndrome

Investigations

- Chromosomes
- Bone age (left wrist X-ray)
- Basal and stimulated gonadotrophin hormone levels
- Early morning testosterone levels
- Thyroid function testing

Treatment

- High-dose testosterone, ideally before stature is excessive

Thalassaemia

> **Comment on this lad's appearance and proceed with any further examination you think appropriate**
>
> Michael is a 15-year-old boy of Mediterranean extraction. He is *pale* and *asthenic*, but otherwise looks well and has no cardio-respiratory distress. He has a number of small scars on the back of his hands and in the ante-cubital fossae, presumably from previous peripheral vein cannulations. He appears *short* for his age and this requires accurate plotting on the appropriate centile chart. On general inspection of his chest and abdomen I note that he has a Porto-cath in situ over the left side of his chest wall. He has multiple small scars on his anterior abdominal wall (from previous desferrioxamine infusions). He has non-tender *splenomegaly* of 6 cm below the right subcostal margin and I can also just palpate the edge of the liver below the left subcostal margin. Michael has a haemoglobinopathy, the most likely being β-*thalassaemia*.

Notes

- The thalassaemias are a family of inherited disorders of haemoglobin synthesis (α chain = chromosome 16, β chain = chromosome 11)
- Most commonly found in the Mediterranean, the Middle East, the Indian subcontinent and southeast Asia
- Carrier status confers protection against the consequences of infection with *Plasmodium falciparum* malaria
- Adult haemoglobin (HbA) = $\alpha_2\beta_2$, fetal haemoglobin = $\alpha_2\gamma_2$, haemoglobin A_2 = $\alpha_2\delta_2$
- Normally Hb A_2 and HbF values should be no higher than 2.5% and 2% of total haemoglobin respectively, after the first 3 years of life. With β-*thalassaemia* major and trait Hb A_2 reaches about 5%. HbF accounts for 60–90% of total haemoglobin in β-*thalassaemia* major and may or may not be elevated with the thalassaemia trait
- The mean cell volume and mean cell haemoglobin are both reduced in β-*thalassaemia* major and trait.
- Presentation of β-*thalassaemia* major is usually in the first year of life with anaemia, poor feeding and abdominal distension (splenomegaly) unless screening has taken place
- If untreated, chronic haemolysis and ineffective erythropoeisis causes gross marrow hyperplasia and extramedullary erythropoesis
- Treatment consists of regular blood transfusions (hypertransfusion

programme) to switch off extramedullary erythropoesis, iron chelation therapy, vitamin C ± folic acid. Iron chelation therapy involves overnight subcutaneous infusions of desferrioxamine, 5–6 nights a week. Oral preparations do exist (deferiprone) but have significant side-effects – neutropenia and arthropathy in 5%. Bone marrow transplantation is curative

- Haemosiderosis of the lymph nodes, adrenals, myocardium, kidneys, pituitary, pancreas and liver causes death in adolescence or early adult life without treatment

Thyroglossal cyst

Examine this girl's neck

On inspection, this girl has a *rounded* swelling in the midline *between the hyoid bone and the suprasternal notch*. It is *fluctuant, smooth and painless* on palpation from behind. On swallowing and sticking out her tongue it moves upwards. She has a *thyroglossal cyst*.

Notes

- Commonest congenital neck swelling
- The thyroid gland develops as a midline outgrowth of cells from the foramen caecum at the base of the tongue. It descends in front of the pharyngeal gut and hyoid bone and normally remains attached to the tongue by the thyroglossal duct that usually obliterates
- Thyroglossal cysts may occur anywhere along the course of the thyroglossal duct
- Occasionally transilluminate
- The cysts can become infected and have a discharging sinus lateral to the midline

Treatment

- Surgical removal
  - cosmetic appearance
  - avoid recurrent infections
  - involves removal of the cyst and hyoid bone and the whole of the thyroglossal duct up to the foramen caecum at the base of the tongue

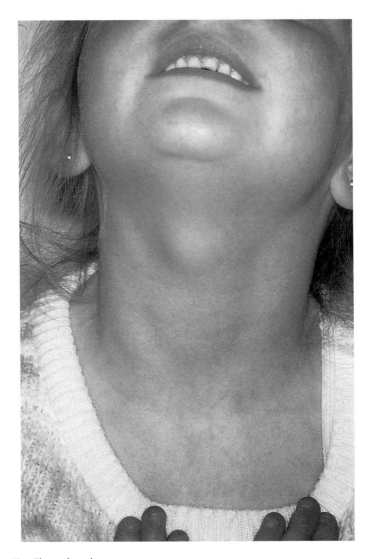

Fig. 43 Thyroglossal cyst

Thyroid goitre

Assess this child's thyroid status

This *thin, restless* young lady is *flushed,* has *warm, sweaty hands* and a *fine tremor* (place a piece of A4 paper on the back of outstretched hands to accentuate this sign). She has *exophthalmos* (look down from above her head to demonstrate this, occurs as a result of lymphocytic infiltration of the retro-orbital tissues), *lid retraction* (due to sympathetic over-stimulation) and upper *lid lag* on downward gaze. Examination of the neck (from behind) reveals *non-tender diffuse swelling* each side of the midline but with no obvious extension retro-sternally (feeling in the supra-sternal notch). The swelling moves upwards with swallowing but not with protruding the tongue (see thyroglossal cyst – page 211). On auscultation a *bruit* can be heard over the swelling. Other evidence to corroborate the diagnosis of *thyrotoxicosis* include a resting heart rate of 120 bpm, *elevated blood pressure* and *increased pulse pressure.* The patient may give a history of weight loss despite an *increased appetite, diarrhoea* and *emotional lability.*

Notes

- Hyperthyroidism in children is almost always due to diffuse toxic goitre (Graves' disease)
- Association with HLA-DR3 and HLA-B8 and other autoimmune disorders (IDDM, coeliac disease, myasthenia gravis)
- Thyroid follicular cell TSH receptor IgG antibodies stimulate thyroid hormone release
- Neonatal thyrotoxicosis occurs as a result of trans-placental passage of thyroid-stimulating immunoglobulin
- Other features: accelerated growth, advanced bone age, proximal muscle weakness, ophthalmoplegia
- Treatment options include anti-thyroid drugs (carbimazole and propylthiouracil), subtotal thyroidectomy and radioactive iodine. Carbimazole is the favoured initial treatment in the UK for children with thyrotoxicosis

Differential diagnosis

- Graves' disease
- Hashimoto's thyroiditis
- Thyroid neoplasm

- Thyroxine poisoning (deliberate or Munchausen syndrome by proxy)
- Pubertal goitre (euthyroid)

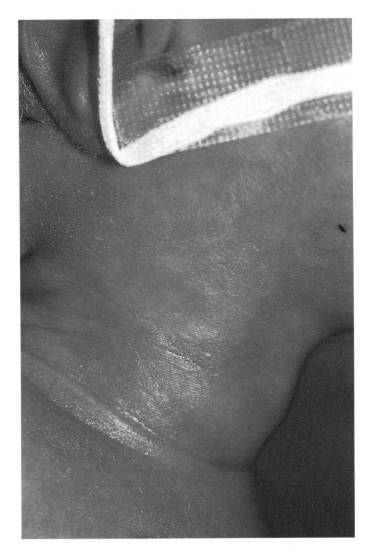

Fig. 44 Transient neonatal hyperthyroidism (and thyroid enlargement) secondary to maternal hyperthyroidism

Treacher Collins' syndrome

What is the diagnosis (spot diagnosis)?

This young lad has the facial features consistent with *Treacher Collins' syndrome* (mandibulofacial dysostosis). He has symmetrically *dysplastic ears* and *hypoplasia* of his *mid-face and mandible*. His palpebral fissures are down-sloping laterally. Looking in his mouth he has a plate in situ for presumed *cleft palate* and he has bilateral *colobomata* of the eyelids. I note that he has bilateral hearing aids (*sensorineural deafness*). His arms appear normal.

Notes

- Autosomal dominant inheritance
- Chromosome 5

Features

- Auricular tags and absent auditory canals
- Absent or sparse eyelashes
- Cardiac defects
- Tracheo-oesophageal fistula

Differential diagnosis

- Goldenhar syndrome – see coloboma (page 65)
- Nager's syndrome (acrofacial dysostosis) – very similar facial appearances, but associated radial limb defects. Autosomal dominant and recessive inheritance reported

Tremor (Wilson's disease)

What are your thoughts on this adolescent's hands?

Simon is a 16-year-old who demonstrates several signs. He has *palmar erythema* and several *spider naevi* on the back of his hands. He also has an *intention tremor* (cerebellar sign, demonstrated by getting him to put both index fingers to either side of the nose, as close as possible without touching it). Looking more widely I note that he has a tinge of *jaundice* – I would like to examine his abdomen for evidence of *hepatosplenomegaly* and *ascites*. Demonstrable extra pyramidal signs include the presence of a *tic*, which Simon has, *rigidity* and *dyskinesia* (*choreoathetosis, bradykinesia, hemiballismus*). Simon also has a degree of *dysarthria* (ask him to tell you his name and address). The combination of hepatic disease and neurological signs suggest *Wilson's disease*.

Notes

- Uncommon autosomal recessive disorder, affecting 1 in 100 000 of the population
- Due to excessive deposition of copper in the cornea (Kayser–Fleischer ring – seen best by slit lamp examination), liver (→ cirrhosis) and basal ganglia (→extra pyramidal signs)
- The primary biochemical abnormality resulting in the defect of copper metabolism and excretion is not known

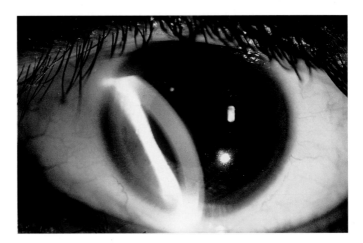

Fig. 45 Kayser–Fleischer ring

- Presents in childhood with liver disease (jaundice, lethargy, abdominal pain), anaemia (haemolytic), portal hypertension (bleeding varices), intellectual and behavioural deterioration, psychiatric disturbance and extrapyramidal signs
- Renal copper deposition can cause Fanconi's syndrome (aminoaciduria) and renal failure. Hypoparathyroidism and arthritis have also been described

Investigations

- Serum caerulopasmin ($\downarrow$)
- Serum copper ($\downarrow$)
- Urine copper excretion ($\uparrow$) especially after penicillamine
- Liver biopsy (copper levels $\uparrow\uparrow$)

Treatment

- D-penicillamine or trientine to chelate copper
- Low copper diet
- Vitamin B$_6$ supplements
- Transplantation if liver failure

Other conditions resulting in extra-pyramidal signs:

- Gilles de la Tourette's syndrome
- Sub-acute sclerosing pan-encephalitis
- Sydenham's chorea
- Heavy metal poisoning
- Ataxia telangiectasia (see page 42)
- Lesch–Nyhan syndrome
  . . . and many others

Involuntary movements

Tremors
- Static tremor – Wilson's, Parkinson's and Huntington's diseases
- Postural tremor – thyrotoxicosis, phaeochromocytoma, physiological
- Intention tremor – Wilson's disease, cerebellar disease

Chorea
- Irregular and rapid movements due to damage in the corpus striatum
- Seen in cerebral palsy (CP), Wilson's disease, Sydenham's chorea, SLE, Lesch–Nyhan disease, PKU, Moyamoya disease

Athetosis
- Slow, writhing movements due to damage to the putamen
- Seen in CP, Wilson's disease, Lesch–Nyhan disease, ataxia telangiectasia

Dystonia
- Sustained abnormal posturing
- Seen in Wilson's disease, drug-induced, Huntington's disease

Myoclonus

- Sudden, irregular contraction of a muscle
- Seen in infantile spasms, myoclonic seizures, Wilson's disease, Tay–Sachs disease, brain infections, CVAs

Tuberous sclerosis

What do you think about this boy's facial skin rash?

This 15-year-old boy has the facial skin appearances of *adenoma sebaceum* with the typical butterfly distribution. Further examination of his skin reveals a number of *hypopigmented areas* on his trunk (which are more easily visualised under Wood's light) and the classical *shagreen patch* over the lumbar region of his spine. He has several *peri-ungual fibromata* on his fingers and toes.

Further examination to confirm the diagnosis of *tuberous sclerosis* (TS) would include measurement of his occipito-frontal head circumference (macrocephaly, secondary to hydrocephalus), retinal examination (*retinal phakoma*), cardiovascular examination (*rhabdomyoma*) and a full developmental assessment.

Notes
- Autosomal dominant inheritance, although up to 90% are new mutations
- Chromosome 9

Presentation
- Skin
  - hypopigmented macules usually present at birth
  - adenoma sebaceum rarely seen before age 2, 50% age 5 years, virtually 100% by 35 years
  - *café au lait* spots and vascular naevi seen more commonly than expected in TS
- Hair – poliosis, a lock of pale hair, can be present at birth.
- CNS
  - infantile spasms
  - developmental delay or regression (40%)
  - epilepsy (60%)
  - hydrocephalus secondary to 'tubers' or malignant change within these (astrocytoma)
- Nails – peri-ungual fibromata
- Kidneys – polycystic disease (80%), angiomyolipomata
- Heart – rhabdomyomata which can result in hydrops fetalis, heart failure, arrhythmia and the Wolff–Parkinson–White syndrome
- Rarely – hamartomas of the lungs ($\rightarrow$ pneumothorax), thyroid, liver, adrenals

Investigations

- EEG – hypsarrhythmia with infantile spasms
- Skull X-ray/CT scan of the brain for tubers ± calcification
- Echocardiography
- Renal ultrasound scan

N.B. Parents should be examined for stigmata of TS and screened with CT scan, echocardiography and renal USS.

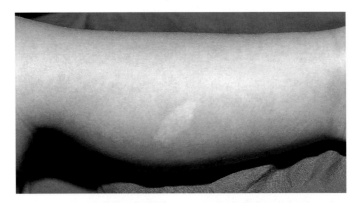

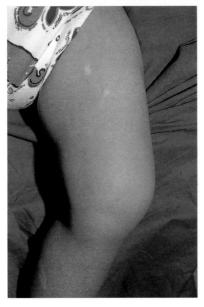

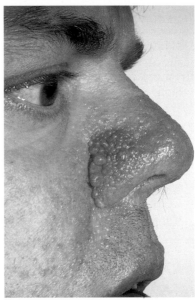

Figs 46–47   Typical hypopigmented macules seen in tuberous sclerosis

Fig 48   Adenoma sebaceum

Turner's syndrome (XO syndrome)

Comment on this girl's appearance

This girl is *short* and I would confirm this by plotting her on an appropriate growth chart. She has a *short, broad, webbed neck* (*pterygium coli*) and a *low posterior hairline*. Her chest is *square-shaped* (shield chest) with *widely spaced nipples*. There are numerous *pigmented naevi* over her chest. She has an increased carrying angle at her elbows (*cubitus valgus*) and *short 4th metacarpals* and *hypoplastic fingernails*. The diagnosis is *Turner's syndrome* and I would like to perform a cardiovascular examination to exclude *coarctation of the aorta*.

Notes

- Incidence = 1 : 7500 girls
- 50% are 45XO; the remainder have altered X chromosome or are mosaic, e.g. 45X/46XX, 45X/46XY, 45X/47XXX
- Approximately 95% of fetuses with 45XO are spontaneously aborted
- 20% of spontaneous abortions have a Turner's karyotype
- Risk of having a girl with Turner's does not increase with increasing maternal age
- Affected girls can be affected with X-linked recessive disorders, e.g. haemophilia A, red-green colour blindness
- Newborn affected infants have low birth weight, lymphoedema of hands and feet and increased nuchal swelling, which can be detected on antenatal ultrasound scans
- Normal life span
- Growth is normal until age 4 when the ovaries involute
- Untreated, the final height is less than 150 cm

Features

- Ovarian dysgenesis (95%)
  - pelvis scan – streak ovaries
  - primary amenorrhoea and failure of development of secondary sexual characteristics
  - basal LH and FSH are high
- Deafness (50%) – secondary to secretory otitis media
- Renal anomalies (40%)
  - horseshoe kidneys
  - duplex ureters
  - normal renal function

- Cardiac anomalies (20%) – coarctation of aorta, aortic stenosis, bicuspid aortic valve
- Increased tendency to keloid scarring
- High arched palate
- Epicanthic folds
- Hypertelorism
- Low average IQ. 10% developmentally delayed
- Prominent ears
- Ptosis
- Micrognathia
- Increased incidence of autoimmune diseases (hypothyroidism)

Differential diagnosis

Noonan's syndrome
- Incidence = 1 : 1500 males = females
- 50% are familial (autosomal dominant)

Features
- Ptosis
- Epicanthic folds
- Low rotated ears
- Down-slanting palpebral fissures
- Hypertelorism
- Short webbed neck
- Low posterior hairline
- Males: cryptorchidism
- Females: delayed puberty
- Congenital heart disease in > 70% (coarctation, pulmonary valve stenosis, hypertrophic cardiomyopathy)
- Short stature
- Cubitus valgus
- Lymphoedema
- Mild learning difficulties (10%)
- Deficiency of factors XI:C, XII:C, VIII:C

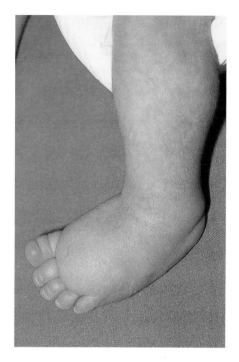

Fig. 49 Neonatal lymphoedema of the feet

Umbilical hernia

Examine this boy's umbilicus

This boy of Afro-Caribbean extraction has a protuberance from his umbilicus. On examination the base of the defect is 1 cm in diameter and the mass originates from the umbilicus. The contents are easily reducible and more demonstrable on standing. The diagnosis is *umbilical hernia*.

Notes

Aetiology
- Physiological – especially common in African children – 40% of black children aged < 1 year have an umbilical hernia
- Prematurity
- Hypothyroidism
- Down's syndrome – see page 88
- Beckwith–Wiederman syndrome – see page 145
- Mucopolysaccharidoses (Hurler's syndrome – see page 123)
- Trisomy 13
- Most umbilical hernias spontaneously regress if the fascial defect is < 1 cm in diameter
- Larger defects may also regress

Indications for surgery
- Incarcination at any age
- Defect > 1.5 cm at 2 years old
- Defect in school-age child

The use of trusses, harnesses and other artificial methods of reducing the hernia do not promote the healing process.

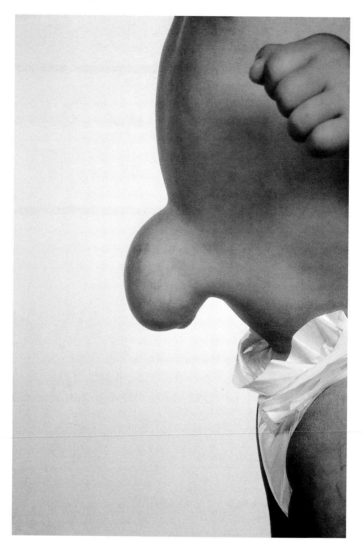

Fig. 50   Umbilical hernia

Undescended testis

Examine this boy's scrotum

On inspection, this young boy has a *hypoplastic, underdeveloped scrotum* on the right. I am unable to palpate the right testis within the scrotum or in the inguinal canal. The left testis is in the scrotum and appears normal. The diagnosis is *right undescended testis*.

Notes

- Incidence
  - full-term newborn – 3.2%
  - 1 year old – 0.7%
- By 1 year old, 80% of *undescended testis* have descended to the scrotum
- No spontaneous testicular descent occurs after 1 year

Full examination of scrotum, perineum needed. Most undescended testis found lateral to the external inguinal ring. Must exclude retractile testes (warm hands necessary!).

Undescended testis
- Associated with inguinal hernia
- Increased risk of torsion
- Increased risk of malignant change
- Infertility in adulthood
- Psychological effects
- Normal histology at birth
- Atrophy at 1 year old
- 30% will develop malignant tumour (aged 30–40)

Bilateral cryptorchidism
- Seen in 30% of cases
- Must check chromosomes
- Usually due to endocrine abnormality at pituitary or testicular level.

Early scrotal placement of undescended testis (within the 1st year of life) is important to decrease the incidence of torsion and traumatic damage. It also improves the prospects of fertility and allows easier examination (for malignant change). However, despite scrotal placement, unde-scended testis remain abnormal, spermatogenesis is rare and there is still an increased risk of malignancy (seminoma).

Ventricular septal defect

Examine this girl's cardiovascular system

This 6-month-old infant is pink in air, but tachypnoeic with a respiratory rate of 40 breaths per minute and mild intercostal and subcostal recession. She is pale and sweaty but has no finger clubbing. Heart rate is 140 beats per minute, of normal volume and character. The apex beat is displaced to the 6th intercostal space in the mid-clavicular line and is thrusting. There is a prominent sternum, visible cardiac pulsation and a left parasternal heave (biventricular hypertrophy). Auscultation reveals a normal 1st heart sound, but the 2nd is obliterated by a harsh pansystolic murmur heard loudest over the lower left sternal edge with radiation throughout the praecordium. This infant also has a 3 cm smooth hepatomegaly. I would complete my examination by measuring the blood pressure and plotting weight and length on the appropriate centile chart for evidence of failure to thrive. This infant has a significant *ventricular septal defect* with evidence of heart failure.

Notes

- Commonest congenital heart malformation (25%)
- An isolated VSD may have a mid-diastolic murmur present as a result of high flow across the mitral valve

Investigations

- CXR – cardiomegaly, prominent pulmonary artery
- ECG – biventricular hypertrophy, notched (left atrium) or peaked (right atrium) P waves
- Echocardiography
- Ventriculography

Treatment

Up to 50% of VSDs will close spontaneously in the first year of life. Of those that do not, a significant number will be asymptomatic. In those that develop heart failure or fail to thrive, diuretics can be tried but surgical intervention should not be a last resort.

Pulmonary artery banding followed by definitive closure after infancy is advocated.

Prophylactic antibiotics against bacterial endocarditis during dental work, genito-urinary and bowel instrumentation and surgery are indicated.

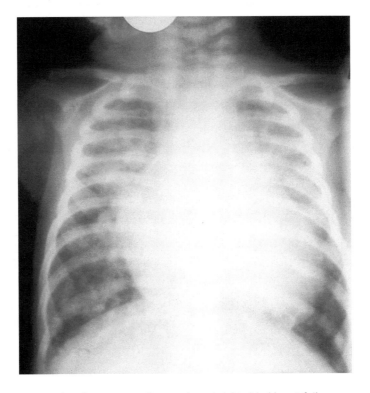

Fig. 51 X-ray showing gross cardiomegaly and right-sided heart failure

Ventriculo-peritoneal shunt

Examine this boy's neck

On examining this 2-year-old boy's neck I can feel a *shunt* with a reservoir, situated at the base of his skull posteriorly. This is most likely to be a *ventriculo-peritoneal shunt*. The boy looks clinically well and has no dysmorphic features. Maximal occipito-frontal head circumference is 54 cm. His posture when sitting (with support) is that of a *flaccid paralysis* of the lower limbs. He has external rotation at the hips, flexion of the knees and plantar flexion at the ankles (the *frog leg* position). He is *areflexic* in his lower limbs and has marked *muscle wasting* and *decreased tone*. Examining his back, there has been surgical intervention, I suspect from closure of a *spina bifida* defect affecting the thoraco-lumbar spine. I would like to go on and formally assess the level of the motor and sensory loss. I note a small surgical transverse incision on the anterior abdominal wall, presumably from placement of the distal portion of the V–P shunt. He does not have any gum hyperplasia (seen with phenytoin).

Notes

- Look for signs of hydrocephalus – sun-setting eyes, squint, macrocephaly, dilated scalp veins, shiny skin, shunt scar. If present, try to transilluminate with a bright torch
- A developmental examination may be asked of you, but if not at least comment on the child's development from observation only and say that you would like to carry out a formal developmental assessment

Causes of hydrocephalus include:
- Prematurity – intraventricular haemorrhage – look for evidence of a 'graduate of the neonatal unit' including scars from venous and arterial cannulation and repeated heel pricks, diplegia or hemiplegia, decreased visual acuity from retinopathy of prematurity
- Spina bifida – as above
- Aqueductal stenosis
- Dandy–Walker cyst – obstruction to the outflow of the IVth ventricle
- Mass lesions – interrupting the flow of cerebrospinal fluid, e.g. tumour, cyst, vein of Galen, haematomas

Normal flow of CSF – produced by the choroid plexus and capillary endothelium of the brain parenchyma. Flows from the lateral ventricle through the foramen of Monro to the IIIrd ventricle. From here through the aqueduct of Sylvius to the IVth ventricle and on into the basal cisterna and cerebral hemispheres via the foramina of Luschka and Magendie.

William's syndrome

What are your thoughts about this young lady?

Anna is a 5-year-old girl who is very *sociable* and enjoys playing with others. She has a *triangular-shaped face* with *prominent lips* and cheeks, *hypertelorism* and *low set ears*. Her head circumference is 44 cm, which I think will be below the 3rd centile for her age when plotted on the appropriate charts. She is also short and again this needs plotting. Developmentally, Anna's speech is difficult to comprehend ('*cocktail party*' *speech*) and I note that she never seems to sit still for very long to concentrate on any one thing. I would now like to go on and examine her cardiovascular system, including blood pressure measurement (hoping to find a *supravalvular aortic stenosis, peripheral pulmonary artery stenosis* or *pulmonary valve stenosis*). Formal developmental assessment is also necessary (say it only if you are slick at developmental assessments and want to be asked to do it!).

I think this young lady has *William's syndrome* with e.g. supravalvular aortic stenosis. I would like to know what her serum calcium, phosphate and alkaline phosphatase are ($\uparrow$, N and $\downarrow$ respectively prior to treatment).

Notes

- William's syndrome is uncommon (incidence 1 in 10 000), but seems to crop up in the short cases with alarming regularity (3 short cases in one – spot diagnosis, cardiovascular exam and developmental assessment)
- It is associated with idiopathic hypercalcaemia, but not always
- Majority are sporadic but autosomal dominant inheritance has been reported (chromosome 7 – disruption of the elastin gene).

Features

- Hypoplastic nails
- Renal artery stenosis
- Dentition abnormalities
- Radio-ulnar synostosis
- Pigmentary abnormalities of the iris
- 'Open mouth' appearance

If asked to perform a developmental assessment in a 5-year-old, don't panic. Comment on general appearance including dysmorphic features, behaviour, growth parameters and any obvious deformities.

Vision and hearing are next – observe what the child does with toys and, if they are willing, give them a piece of paper and pencil to draw something. By asking them to draw 'mummy' you are assessing hearing, understanding and their fine motor skills. If problems of cooperation, try drawing something yourself and hopefully they will imitate you. Formal audiology is necessary if doubts arise about abilities to hear properly (although you will not be in the ideal situation to assess anything appropriately in the RCPCH/DCH short case exam!).

Fine motor skills are being assessed during the previous section. Add to this by getting them to thread beads onto a piece of string or put a pen top onto the pen.

Gross motor skills can be assessed by getting the child to walk and run, skip, hop, climb onto a chair and stand on one leg or the other.

During this process you should have observed behaviour, sociability, language and speech and interactions with others.

Refer to Table 1 in the developmental assessment section (page 29) for a very basic list of developmental milestones. At least know these off by heart.

Index and differential diagnosis